EMS Response
to Patients with Special Needs

EMS Response
to Patients with Special Needs

Assessment, Treatment, and Transport

Katherine Koch

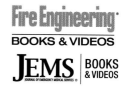

Fire Engineering

BOOKS & VIDEOS

JEMS | **BOOKS & VIDEOS**

JOURNAL OF EMERGENCY MEDICAL SERVICES ®

Disclaimer

The recommendations, advice, descriptions, and methods in this book are presented solely for educational purposes. The author and publisher assume no liability whatsoever for any loss or damage that results from the use of any of the material in this book. Use of the material in this book is solely at the risk of the user.

Copyright © 2020 by
Fire Engineering Books & Videos
110 S. Hartford Ave., Suite 200
Tulsa, Oklahoma 74120 USA

800.752.9764
+1.918.831.9421
info@fireengineeringbooks.com
www.FireEngineeringBooks.com

Senior Vice President: Eric Schlett
Operations Manager: Holly Fournier
Sales Manager: Joshua Neal
Managing Editor: Mark Haugh
Production Manager: Tony Quinn
Developmental Editor: Chris Barton
Book Designer: Susan E. Ormston
Cover Designer: Brandon Ash
Indexer: Sophia R. Purut

Library of Congress Cataloging-in-Publication Data Available on Request

ISBN: 978-1-59370-498-8
eISBN: 978-1-59370-852-8

Printed in the United States of America

1 2 3 4 5   24 23 22 21 20

Contents

Preface

This book came about through an unexpected meeting of my two careers. I had been a classroom special education teacher for 10 years before moving to the college classroom, teaching future teachers about working with K–12 students with disabilities. I also obtained my National Registry Paramedic certification and state license after being a volunteer EMT for several years. I realized there was a gap in the literature regarding people with medical and traumatic emergencies who also had a cognitive, physical, or medical disability. Both my EMT and paramedic training lacked guidelines for working with patients with disabilities, save for a few brief mentions in the "special populations" chapters of my textbooks. I realized that a large subset of our population could be at risk for misunderstandings, potentially inadequate patient care, and incorrect or even dangerous interventions due to insufficient knowledge about disabilities in general and the issues particular to specific disabilities.

This is not new. For centuries, people with cognitive, physical, and medical disabilities often received incorrect care, no care at all, or were institutionalized. People with disabilities were often involuntarily placed in crowded, dirty, and unregulated facilities. Women with disabilities were sterilized against their will.[1] Between 1907 and 1937, more than 58,000 people in 29 states, mostly women, were sterilized on the basis of having a cognitive impairment ("feebleminded"), insanity, seizures, tuberculosis, syphilis, blindness, deafness, and/or physical impairments, as well as others considered "socially inadequate," including gay and lesbian people, the homeless, orphans, and drug users.[2] In 1927 forced sterilization of those with disabilities was legalized by the US Supreme Court in the case *Buck v. Bell*. This ruling has never been overturned by the courts and remains in place today.

In the latter half of the 19th century, some major cities, including San Francisco and Chicago, passed laws that actually banned people with disabilities, including returning injured and maimed Civil War veterans, from being seen in public.[3] These laws, known as the "ugly laws," were first passed in San Francisco in 1867 to reduce street begging by those with disabilities. Passed in 1881, the Chicago ordinance stated:

> Any person who is diseased, maimed, mutilated, or in any way deformed, so as to be an unsightly or disgusting object, or an improper

person to be allowed in or on the streets, highways, thoroughfares, or public places in the city, shall not therein or thereon expose himself to public view, under the penalty of a fine of $1 for each offense.[4]

These laws included a vast array of disabilities and were intended to prevent these so-called undesirables from negatively impacting public life. Epilepsy was considered so disturbing that it was assumed that someone observing another person having a seizure would be forever haunted by the experience.[5] There were similar "ugly laws" across the country that were not repealed until the latter half of the 20th century. Chicago's law was finally repealed in 1973.

In the early years of the 20th century, immigrants to the United States arriving at Ellis Island were subjected to intrusive and undignified physical exams. Those with disabilities who were found to be "defectives and undesirables"[6] were refused entry to the United States and were deported back to their home countries. It was feared that people with cognitive, mental health, and physical disabilities would be unable to work and therefore would become the responsibility of the government. Even those who could clearly demonstrate that they had been supporting themselves financially and were able to continue doing so were typically denied entrance.[7]

Due to this overall lack of support, families were often unable to care for their relatives with disabilities and usually would turn them over to the care of the state.[8] Even today, people with disabilities are at a higher risk of death. While some of those deaths are directly related to the individuals' disabilities, some are not clearly attributable and have no explanation.[9]

As time progressed, however, the rights of those with disabilities began to be considered, and through legislation, improved. There are now several laws that support the rights of those with disabilities.[10]

- **Architectural Barriers Act (42 U.S.C. §§ 4151 et seq.) (1968).** Requires that all buildings that are "designed, constructed, or altered with Federal funds" be accessible to people with disabilities.

- **Section 504 of the Rehabilitation Act (29 U.S.C. § 794) (1973).** States that no person with a disability "shall be excluded from, denied the benefits of, or be subjected to discrimination" under any program that receives federal funding. This act also requires schools and employers to provide reasonable accommodations for students and employees with disabilities.

- **Individuals with Disabilities Education Act (20 U.S.C. §§ 1400 et seq.) (1975).** Requires public schools to make education accessible and appropriate for children with disabilities.

- **Civil Rights of Institutionalized Persons Act (42 U.S.C. §§ 1997 et seq.) (1980).** Authorizes the US Attorney General to investigate conditions at institutions such as prisons, detention centers, and nursing homes, as well as institutions for people with developmental or psychiatric disabilities. This act is designed to protect the health and safety of people living in these institutions.

- **Fair Housing Act (42 U.S.C. §§ 3601 et seq.) (1988).** Requires landlords to make reasonable exceptions to their policies to allow people with disabilities equal housing opportunities. This can include relaxing a no-pet policy to allow for service dogs and allowing tenants to make minor modifications to increase access. New multi-family (four or more units) construction is required to be designed and built to accommodate access.

- **Americans with Disabilities Act (42 U.S.C. §§ 12101 et seq.) (1990).** Prohibits discrimination in employment, government activities, public buildings, transportation, and television/telephone access. See more discussion of the ADA in chapter 1.

Unfortunately, laws do not guarantee understanding of the issues experienced by people with disabilities, nor do they guarantee that discrimination, inadvertent or deliberate, will not happen. The lingering effects of decades of limited acknowledgment of the medical needs of people with disabilities are seen in healthcare disparities today.[11] Insurance coverage is often inadequate for comprehensive treatment of developmental disabilities such as autism spectrum disorders, intellectual disabilities, and emotional or mental health disorders. People with disabilities often live with less education, less money, less internet access, and fewer transportation options. These factors often lead to unhealthy lifestyles, poorer physical and mental health, and a greater need for health care combined with a greater difficulty accessing it.[12]

The potential for discrimination and a lack of understanding are also seen with medical practitioners, both in and out of hospital settings. The lack of training and knowledge is chiefly to blame.[13]

Twenty-two family physicians were interviewed about their comfort level in working with patients with intellectual disabilities (ID). All of the participants in this study reported that they were not sufficiently prepared to work with patients with ID, even those who were primarily working with patients with ID by choice. The concerns that emerged from the interviews with these practicing physicians were 1) a lack of knowledge about ID, 2) lack of confidence with interacting with these patients, especially with communication and dealing with challenging behaviors, and 3) not being familiar with the daily lives of their patients and the implications for providing medical care. All the physicians reported that they would have liked to have had the care of people with ID incorporated into their medical school curriculum.[14]

A recent smaller study looked at the attitudes of medical students as they prepared to become physicians.[15] Some of the students who were interviewed had positive comments on learning about and working with this population in the future. Others reported they did not feel that having content on ID in their medical school curriculum was necessary, even though they had concerns about working with this population. There were also overall concerns about feeling anxious working with people who have ID and the lack of knowledge needed to be effective practitioners.

One study that reviewed the previous training and current knowledge of 256 psychiatrists related to working with patients with ID revealed similar concerns. More than 90% reported that they did not have adequate training in the identification and treatment of people with ID but agreed that training in this area was important.[16]

The results of these studies highlight the need for improved physician education related to treating people with ID. And while ID is only one type of disability, no literature was found to show that healthcare providers are any better educated and prepared to address other disabilities.

The focus of this book, however, is prehospital emergency medicine and disabilities, an area where knowledge and understanding are even more limited. It is my hope that this text will start a larger discussion about the need to include disability education in EMT and paramedic curricula.

The information presented in this book is for educational purposes only and is not intended to supplant your local or state protocols. As always, remember to contact medical control with any questions or concerns about a course of treatment.

Acknowledgments

This book would not have been possible without the support of my husband (and fellow paramedic) Paul, as he loved and supported me while writing and revising and covering every flat surface in the house with reference books and articles.

Additional thanks to my children, Andrew, Abigail, and Molly, all dedicated EMS providers. (We can staff an entire ambulance just with family.) They are everything to me.

Special thanks to Betty Raines Azwell for her helpful and thorough edits, to all the children with disabilities I had the privilege to teach, and to my patients from whom I learn so much by caring for them.

Notes

1. Kim E. Nielsen, *A Disability History of the United States* (Boston: Beacon Press, 2012); and Gloria L. Krahn, Deborah K. Walker, and Rosaly Correa-De-Araujo, "Persons with Disabilities as an Unrecognized Health Disparity Population," *American Journal of Public Health* 105, no. S2 (2015): S198–S206, https://doi.org/10.2105/ajph.2014.302182.

2. Nielsen, *A Disability History of the United States*, 115.

3. Susan M. Schweik, *The Ugly Laws: Disability in Public* (New York: New York University, 2009); and Nielsen, *A Disability History of the United States*.

4. Schweik, *The Ugly Laws*, 1.

5. Schweik, *The Ugly Laws*.

6. Nielsen, *A Disability History of the United States*, 107.

7. Nielsen, *A Disability History of the United States*.

8. Perri Meldon, "Disability History: Early and Shifting Attitudes of Treatment," US Department of the Interior, National Park Service, retrieved May 30, 2018, https://www.nps.gov/articles/disabilityhistoryearlytreatment.htm.

9. Istvan M. Majer et al., "Mortality Risk Associated with Disability: A Population-Based Record Linkage Study," *American Journal of Public Health* 101, no. 12 (2011): E9–E15, https://doi.org/10.2105/ajph.2011.300361.

10. US Department of Justice, Civil Rights Division, Disability Rights Section, *A Guide to Disability Rights* (US Department of Justice, July 2009), https://www.ada.gov/cguide.htm.

11. Krahn, Walker, and Correa-De-Araujo, "Persons with Disabilities as an Unrecognized Health Disparity Population."

12. Krahn, Walker, and Correa-De-Araujo, "Persons with Disabilities as an Unrecognized Health Disparity Population."

13. Mhairi Duff, Matt Hoghton, and Mark Scheepers, "More Training is Needed in Health Care of People with Learning Disabilities," *BMJ* 321, no. 7,257 (2000): 385–386.

14. Joanne Wilkinson et al., "'Sometimes I Feel Overwhelmed': Educational Needs of Family Physicians Caring for People with Intellectual Disabilities," *Intellectual and Developmental Disabilities* 50, no. 3 (2012): 243–250, https://doi.org/10.1352/1934-9556-50.3.243.

15. Travis A. Ryan and Katrina Scior, "Medical Students' Attitudes towards Health Care for People with Intellectual Disabilities: A Qualitative Study," *Journal of Applied Research in Intellectual Disabilities* 29, no. 6 (2015): 508–518, https://doi.org/10.1111/jar.12206.

16. S. Werner et al., "Psychiatrists' Knowledge, Training and Attitudes Regarding the Care of Individuals with Intellectual Disability," *Journal of Intellectual Disability Research* 57, no. 8 (2013): 774–782, https://doi.org/10.1111/j.1365-2788.2012.01604.x.

1

Introduction to Disability: Remember the Basics

You are dispatched as a paramedic chase vehicle to rendezvous with a basic life support (BLS) ambulance on scene with a patient complaining of chest pain. The dispatcher says the patient was on board a van that was transporting participants in an adult day program for people with intellectual disabilities. As you arrive, the EMT is securing the patient to the stretcher. The van driver does not have any information about the patient but says that he will contact the program coordinator to let her know that the patient is going to the hospital. You climb on the ambulance and introduce yourself to the patient. When you ask, she says her name is Phyllis and that she is 48 years old. When you ask her to tell you what is wrong, she simply says, "It hurts here," and points to the middle of her chest.

As you attempt to gain a medical history, you realize that your typical process of asking open-ended questions is not working, as she is not responding. You try a different approach by asking simple, direct questions. Instead of asking, "Do you have any medical problems?" you ask, "Do you have any problems with your heart?" Phyllis responds, "No." Then you ask, "Do you have diabetes?" She says she does. Forgetting the plan to ask simple, direct questions, you ask what she takes to control her diabetes, and you get a confused look in response. Trying again, you ask, "Do you take pills to help with your sugar?" She responds, "Yes, and shots." You continue asking simple questions, and by the time you get to the hospital you have a reasonable history (no cardiac history, but insulin dependent diabetes and GERD) along with a 12-lead EKG and several sets of vitals to give to the triage nurse. You tell her about Phyllis's chief complaint, along with her history. You let the nurse know that Phyllis has trouble answering open-ended or complex questions and suggest the nurse keep her questions and directions short and unambiguous.

According to the 2010 US Census,[1] 56.7 million people (18.7%) over the age of six years report a sensory, communication, physical, mental, or self-care disability. Therefore, it is very likely that EMS providers, firefighters, and law enforcement personnel will encounter a patient with a disability that contributes to, exacerbates, or complicates a medical or traumatic emergency.

Some highlights from the data include the following:[2]

- The number of people in the United States with a disability increased by 2.2 million from 2005 to 2010.
- Of adults aged 21 to 64 with a disability, 41% were employed as compared with 79% of adults without disabilities.
- Almost 11% of adults aged 15 to 64 with severe disabilities were likely to experience persistent poverty compared to almost 5% of adults with nonsevere disabilities and almost 4% of adults with no disability.
- Among people greater than 80 years old, 71% reported a disability. Children less than 15 years old had a disability rate of just over 8%.
- In adults aged 15 years and older, 6.2% had some level of difficulty with vision, hearing, or verbal communication.
- Limitations associated with the lower body (e.g., requiring the use of a wheelchair, crutches, or walker) were reported in almost 13% of adults 15 years and older, and 8% reported difficulty with upper body functions (e.g., lifting or grasping).
- Just over 6% of adults had cognitive, mental, or emotional functioning difficulties, including learning disabilities, intellectual disabilities, dementia, and autism spectrum disorders.
- Three percent of adults reported disabling anxiety or depression.

Despite these statistics, cognitive, physical, mental, and sensory disabilities are either not covered or are covered only minimally in EMS training. A review of five prominent EMS textbooks that averaged 49 total chapters and more than 1,400 pages revealed only one chapter each on meeting the needs of patients with special challenges or disabilities. In EMT and paramedic training programs, there is limited formal instruction or information on assessing and treating patients with disabilities, yet EMS providers are expected to care for those with disabilities and their special needs.

Americans with Disabilities Act

The Americans with Disabilities Act (ADA) (table 1–1), a civil rights law enacted in 1990, amended in 2008, and revised in 2010, was established because the US Congress found that individuals with disabilities were being discriminated against in many areas, including healthcare. While some improvements had been made prior to 1990, people with disabilities were still being discriminated against as well as segregated and isolated. Until the passage of the ADA, they had no legal recourse. Therefore, the purpose of the ADA is "to provide a clear and comprehensive national mandate for the elimination of discrimination against individuals with disabilities" and "to provide clear, strong, consistent, enforceable standards addressing discrimination against individuals with disabilities."[3]

Inclusivity of people with disabilities into the community, including into mainstream healthcare, is the moral, ethical, and kind thing to do. It is also the law. And as people with disabilities are more authentically included in the community, rather than hospitalized or institutionalized, prehospital EMS providers will be increasingly likely to encounter a patient with a disability that is either a direct cause of the emergency call or is a complicating factor in the emergency situation.

Table 1–1. Americans with Disabilities Act

TITLE 42 THE PUBLIC HEALTH AND WELFARE
CHAPTER 126 EQUAL OPPORTUNITY FOR INDIVIDUALS WITH DISABILITIES
Sec. 12101. Findings and purpose
(a) Findings.
The Congress finds that
(1) physical or mental disabilities in no way diminish a person's right to fully participate in all aspects of society, yet many people with physical or mental disabilities have been precluded from doing so because of discrimination; others who have a record of a disability or are regarded as having a disability also have been subjected to discrimination;

Table 1–1. ...*continued*

(2) historically, society has tended to isolate and segregate individuals with disabilities, and, despite some improvements, such forms of discrimination against individuals with disabilities continue to be a serious and pervasive social problem;

(3) discrimination against individuals with disabilities persists in such critical areas as employment, housing, public accommodations, education, transportation, communication, recreation, institutionalization, health services, voting, and access to public services;

(4) unlike individuals who have experienced discrimination on the basis of race, color, sex, national origin, religion, or age, individuals who have experienced discrimination on the basis of disability have often had no legal recourse to redress such discrimination;

(5) individuals with disabilities continually encounter various forms of discrimination, including outright intentional exclusion, the discriminatory effects of architectural, transportation, and communication barriers, overprotective rules and policies, failure to make modifications to existing facilities and practices, exclusionary qualification standards and criteria, segregation, and relegation to lesser services, programs, activities, benefits, jobs, or other opportunities;

(6) census data, national polls, and other studies have documented that people with disabilities, as a group, occupy an inferior status in our society, and are severely disadvantaged socially, vocationally, economically, and educationally;

(7) the Nation's proper goals regarding individuals with disabilities are to assure equality of opportunity, full participation, independent living, and economic self-sufficiency for such individuals; and

(8) the continuing existence of unfair and unnecessary discrimination and prejudice denies people with disabilities the opportunity to compete on an equal basis and to pursue those opportunities for which our free society is justifiably famous, and costs the United States billions of dollars in unnecessary expenses resulting from dependency and nonproductivity.

Source: ADA, 42 U.S.C. §12101(a), https://www.ada.gov/pubs/ada.htm.

Access to Medical Care

Despite the ADA providing legislation to protect the rights of those with disabilities, the expectations of the law are not always upheld, as barriers to health care continue to be prevalent in this population.

According to research by Cannoodt et al., barriers to emergency care exist for all people, not just those with disabilities.[4] They include religious or cultural reasons, financial limitations, geographical challenges (living in remote areas, for example), lack of transportation, and language differences. Barriers to access for emergency care may also arise due to limited resources, including understaffed hospitals and lengthy waits in the emergency departments. Although Cannoodt et al. do not specifically identify disability as a barrier to emergency care access, people with disabilities are at a higher risk for experiencing the barriers that they do identify.[5] Common barriers include lack of transportation, limited financial resources, and language challenges (people with disabilities may be nonverbal or may have difficulty communicating what is wrong).

People with disabilities may have additional challenges in maintaining healthy lifestyle practices, also related to their disability.[6] Fatigue, chronic pain, obesity, depression, limited mobility, and poor wheelchair access to transportation and buildings can make it difficult or impossible to exercise, shop for healthy foods, make regular physician visits, and obtain needed prescriptions or other medical supplies. This can exacerbate existing medical conditions associated with the disability and increase the likelihood of a 911 call, either because the individual is having a medical or psychiatric crisis or because they have no other way to access health care except by ambulance.

A 2006 study investigating environmental barriers to health care for people with disabilities reported 22% of those surveyed said they had difficulty accessing a healthcare provider's office due to its location or its office layout.[7] In total, almost 85% of people with disabilities surveyed in this study reported environmental barriers, including social isolation, lack of disability resource information, limited access to healthcare, or unfair treatment by healthcare providers.[8]

A more recent study reveals that barriers continue to be a problem with preventative and ongoing medical care.[9]

- Mobility and cognitive issues reduce access to routine preventative care (e.g., mammograms, pap smears, cholesterol checks, colonoscopies, etc.) and ongoing care for identified health concerns like diabetes and hypertension.

- Chronic illnesses such as diabetes and cardiovascular disease can be as much as five times the rate of the general population.

- There is an increased risk of injury and assault in people with disabilities.

- Depression and anxiety are seen at higher rates.

- Insurance coverage can be inadequate and associated costs (e.g., copays) can be an additional barrier.[10]

As a result of these barriers, emergency department use is high in individuals with disabilities. According to one study, almost 40% of total emergency department visits were made by working adults with a disability despite being only 17% of the adult workforce.[11] Individuals with disabilities had a higher frequency of emergency visits in nearly all illness categories that could precipitate an emergency visit, including hypertension, neck and back pain, psychiatric concerns, heart problems, and respiratory complaints.[12] All patients in this study reported limited access to medical care and prescriptions, but patients with disabilities had much higher rates of limited access than those without disabilities and tended to have more complicated health needs.[13]

Because of their limited access to routine and ongoing health care, along with the increased incidence of medical and psychiatric crises in people with disabilities, a high rate of prehospital emergency services usage should be expected.

Person-First Language

Think about how you like to be addressed. Most people prefer to be called by their given name, a nickname, or a title (Mr., Mrs., Mom, Grandpa, etc.), and not by a descriptive characteristic, particularly a disability characteristic. Sometimes that is not possible (if we do not know the person's name) or practical (the description is important or particularly relevant to the conversation). But considering your use of language as you interact with patients and their families, especially the use of person-first language rather than identity-first language, can go a long way to forming relationships and building trust with them in the short time you are together.

Person-first language means not using the disability to describe the person but recognizing the person is primary before the disability, so the disability is something they *have* instead of something they *are*. Person-first language demonstrates inclusivity and respect for others.[14] The disability, condition, or illness should never be used as an adjective to *describe the person* (e.g., "the autistic person"). Instead it should only be used as a noun when *describing a condition* (e.g., "the person who is autistic"). This means referring to "the person with autism," not "the autistic person" or simply "the autistic." The person comes first, the disability comes second. The Arc of the United States, a national community-based organization that provides support and advocacy for individuals with intellectual and developmental disabilities, notes that person-first language is an "objective way of acknowledging, communicating, and reporting on disabilities. It eliminates generalizations and stereotypes, by focusing on the person rather than the disability."[15]

While this is typically considered the appropriate and standard language usage when referring to people with disabilities, not all those in the disability community prefer person-first language. Some communities would rather be identified with identity-first language. Those in the Deaf community may view themselves as Deaf individuals who are part of a Deaf culture. (Some prefer to use an uppercase D when referring to the culture or community and a lowercase d to refer to the "audiological condition."[16]) We are beginning to see this emerge in the autism community as well. Some disability rights scholars and people with disabilities themselves prefer the use of identity-first language, asserting that it returns ownership of the label to the individual carrying the label[17] and is not something to be viewed as negative or pathological, but merely a nonpejorative description of a normal part of the human condition.

You should also be cautious with word choices that surround the description of the disability. The person does not "suffer from" spina bifida; they "have" spina bifida. They are not a "victim" of dementia; they "live with" or "have" dementia. They are not "wheelchair-bound." They "use a wheelchair for mobility." Using language that has a negative or deficit connotation is demeaning and continues to perpetuate the idea that people with disabilities are somehow less than those without. This is not to say that people with disabilities do not experience challenges and difficulties, but the goal is to recognize that their lives encompass more than the things in their lives that may be difficult.

In a perfect world, we would be able to go through life without labeling (or mislabeling) people based on their physical, mental, or cognitive characteristics. But in real life, and especially when we are providing emergency medical care, knowing about an individual's disability may be critical to their assessment and treatment. How we address a person can also make a difference in how they feel about their care and how they interact with providers. If you are unsure what someone's disability might be, ask them or their caregiver. It can help you decide on appropriate assessment and treatment strategies as well as help establish rapport. (See the next section for more discussion on appropriate communication.)

Because there are those with disabilities who prefer person-first language, and those who prefer identity-first language, it can be impossible for you to initially know the preferred way to speak about the disability around that individual. One way to deal with this is to listen to how they (or their family) describe themselves and follow suit. Does your patient say, "I am autistic," or do they say, "I have autism"? Does the family member say, "My sister is intellectually disabled," or "My sister has an intellectual disability"? You will not go wrong by being respectful and careful in your language choices and defaulting to person-first language unless you are told otherwise (table 1–2).

Table 1–2. Suggestions on language choices to use and to avoid

Say this...	Instead of this...
She has a physical disability.	She is crippled.
	She is handicapped.
He uses a wheelchair.	He is wheelchair bound.
	He is confined to a wheelchair.
She has depression/anxiety.	She has a mental problem.
He has bipolar disorder.	He is bipolar.
She is a child without a disability/with typical development/neurotypical.	She is normal.
He has an intellectual/developmental disability.	He is mentally retarded.
She has a disability.	She is disabled.
He is deaf.	He is hearing impaired.
He is hard of hearing.	

Table 1–2. ...*continued*

She is nonverbal.	She is mute. She is dumb.
He has a seizure disorder.	He is an epileptic.
She has autism.	She is autistic. She is an autistic.
He has Down syndrome.	He is Downs. He is a mongoloid.
She has a congenital disability. She was born with...	She has a birth defect.
He needs an accessible restroom stall.	He needs a handicapped restroom stall.
She lives with...	She is...
He has...	He suffers from... He is afflicted with...

Communication

Some disabilities present with characteristics that make it easy to recognize that the patient has physical or cognitive differences. If your patient uses a wheelchair or crutches for mobility, or displays the classic facial characteristics of Down syndrome, you can safely make some *general* assumptions about their potential special needs during assessment, treatment, and transport. Some disabilities, such as autism, traumatic brain injury, and mental health disorders (depression, anxiety, ADHD, etc.), do not have any outward physical characteristics, and you may not know if the person has a diagnosis unless they tell you.

In the same vein, with some disabilities such as cerebral palsy or autism, it is difficult to know quickly and easily if the person also has an intellectual disability. The characteristics of the primary disability may mask their cognitive abilities. For example, some people with autism do not use their voices to communicate when stressed or ill, and one could then make the erroneous assumption that they also have cognitive difficulties. Some forms of cerebral palsy impact the fine muscles of the mouth. As a result, the person's speech can be slurred or halting, making it hard to understand them. But their problems with the mechanisms of speech do not correlate with cognitive deficits. If you are unsure, assume your patient does not have a cognitive or intellectual disability unless told otherwise. But also expect that some behaviors and language usage might be below age level. There may be no outward signs of a cognitive disability, but the person can have challenges with thinking and oral language.

It is impossible to know exactly how your patient's disability will manifest just by knowing what the disability is. For example, while there are several common characteristics of people with autism, such as impairments in social communication and restricted and repetitive behaviors, how those characteristics manifest in any one individual can vary widely.

Unless your patient is a child, do not treat them like a child, even if they have an intellectual disability. Remember that they are adults and treat them as such. That includes speaking directly to the individual and not talking about and around them with caregivers. But also recognize the value of family and caregivers and use them as assets in your assessment and care. While you may be the expert on prehospital emergency assessment and treatment, they are the expert on that individual and their condition (secondary, of course, to the individual themselves). Use their knowledge to your benefit. This does not mean allowing them to take over the scene, drive your assessment, or insist on a particular treatment. It does mean letting them share what they know that will facilitate your assessment and interventions, and treating them, along with the patient, with respect.

Service and Support Animals

It is becoming more common to see service and support animals in public places. Guide dogs for those who are blind or have limited vision are familiar to most people, but increasingly service animals are being used by people with a wide range of disabilities to more fully participate in everyday life. Animals have been trained for early detection of seizures, hypoglycemia, and panic attacks. Service and support animals may be employed to respond to sounds on behalf of people who are deaf or hard-of-hearing, or they may be used to alert people to the presence of an allergen. Service animals may offer physical support by retrieving items, opening doors, and assisting with mobility and balance. Service and emotional support animals may be used to help those with anxiety disorders and PTSD.

The Americans with Disabilities Act (ADA) defines a service animal as "a dog that is individually trained to do work or perform tasks for a person with a disability."[18] In addition to dogs, the ADA also recognizes, in some cases, miniature horses as an alternative to dogs.[19] In such cases the miniature horse must be trained to support the person with a disability. The size and weight of the miniature horse must be considered, along with the individual's control over the miniature horse and if the miniature horse is housebroken.

The ADA has clear guidelines and expectations for how service animals are to be accommodated, both for the public and for the handler. With very few exceptions, service animals are to be allowed in all public places. An individual with a disability can only be asked to remove their service animal from a public place if the animal is noisy/disruptive, not under sufficient control (harness, leash, voice, or hand signals) of the handler, or if it is not housebroken. If any of these conditions are met, the animal may be removed, but the individual with a disability *must be otherwise accommodated sufficiently to be able to participate in the activity or event.* A fear of or allergy to dogs/horses is not an acceptable reason to deny admittance of a service animal.[20]

Additionally, it is not permitted to ask the handler about why they need the service animal or about what disability they have. The ADA allows two questions to be asked:

1. "Is the animal required because of a disability?"

2. "What work or task has the animal been trained to perform?"

These questions should not be asked if the support the animal is giving is obvious (such as a guide dog for a person who is blind). A license, certification, or other verification that the animal has been trained to perform a task is not required and may not be requested.

There are other general etiquette expectations when interacting with a service animal and its handler. While some of these guidelines may be irrelevant in an emergency situation, they are important to keep in mind nonetheless.

- Do not touch the service animal without permission from the handler. This can be distracting for the animal and the person.
- Do not offer the service animal food, treats, or toys.

- Speak directly to the handler. Do not speak directly to the animal or try to gain its attention by whistling, clapping, or snapping your fingers. In fact, it is entirely appropriate to ignore the animal completely.
- If the person does not appear physically disabled, do not assume that the animal is not a legitimate service animal or that it is not legitimately needed. Many people have "invisible" disabilities but still need support. Speculating or commenting on the legitimacy of a service animal is inappropriate. While there have been many reports of fake service dogs, and indeed there are a plethora of ways to falsify service dog vests and credentials, even if you are concerned about the veracity of a particular animal, it is best to err on the side of the patient and treat it as a legitimate service animal.

Comfort, emotional support, and companion animals do not perform a specific task or skill, so under the ADA requirements, they are not considered service animals. If the animal, however, is able to recognize that a person is experiencing emotional distress and actively intervenes to redirect and calm the person, it may be considered a service animal and must be accommodated.

Questions may arise concerning whether or not ambulance crews are expected to transport a service animal in the ambulance with the patient. Generally the answer is yes if there is room to transport the animal in the ambulance and the animal remains under the control of its handler, even while they are under emergency medical care, and it does not interfere with patient care. Exactly where the service animal sits during transport can depend on the nature of the emergency, the condition of the patient, and the size of the animal. If the transport is fairly routine and the animal is small, it can sit (secured) on the stretcher with the patient. A larger animal might be better accommodated on one of the seats. This would also be appropriate during a transport requiring significant interventions. As with all potential projectiles in a moving vehicle (including people and objects such as monitors and oxygen tanks), the service animal should be safely secured for transport. A variety of commercial leashes and harnesses are available that can be secured with the seatbelts in the ambulance, or the service animal can ride in a kennel.

In cases where there is no room in the ambulance or it is impractical to transport the service animal in the ambulance, alternate arrangements should be made for simultaneous transport of the service animal to the hospital. Depending on the situation, there are several transport options:

- A family member or neighbor can transport the service animal in a private vehicle.
- An EMS/fire supervisor can transport the service animal in the supervisor's vehicle.
- In an area with an advanced life support (ALS) chase car system, the service animal can ride with the person driving the chase car.
- Law enforcement or animal control could provide service animal transport as long as the service animal is not in close proximity to K9 dogs or other animals.

Regardless of what vehicle the service animal is in, it should be secured appropriately for transport for its safety as well as for the people who are transporting the service animal. Remember, this service animal is serving a vital purpose for the patient. Separating the patient from their service animal can be traumatizing and frightening for both human and animal. It may be to your advantage and can ultimately facilitate your patient care to allow the animal to be transported with the patient. While you are not legally obligated to transport a nonservice comfort animal, consider the needs of your patient along with your need to assess and treat appropriately. Allowing the patient to bring their comfort animal may actually facilitate your care. It would be appropriate, however, to remind your patient and their family that the hospital is under no obligation to allow a nonservice comfort animal, so they will want to plan for alternative care upon arrival at the emergency department.

As with any scene or situation, the decision about how and where to transport a service animal should be based on the individual circumstances of the events, patient, and EMS providers. You should be prepared to act as your patient's advocate at the emergency department, if necessary, by reminding the staff that the service animal's presence is protected by federal law.

Wheelchair Etiquette

EMS providers often encounter patients who use mobility assistance devices such as wheelchairs or scooters, either because they are unable to walk, because they have difficulty walking easily or efficiently due to extremity pain or weakness, or because of health conditions that cause general fatigue or weakness. While the specific conditions that may contribute to a person needing to use a wheelchair for mobility assistance are discussed in greater detail in later chapters, here are some general suggestions when interacting with people who use wheelchairs:

- Ask permission before pushing a person's wheelchair, especially if they are in it. Unless it is a situation where you would physically pick up the person and carry them to another location without their consent, do not push them in their wheelchair without their consent. It is essentially the same thing.

- Do not touch, lean on, or grab the wheelchair. It is an extension of their body and personal space.

- If practical and appropriate, sit at the individual's eye level during an extended conversation so they are not looking up at you.

- Speak directly to the individual, not to a caregiver, and in a normal tone and volume of voice (unless you are told they are hearing impaired and need increased volume).

- If they transfer out of the wheelchair, be sure not to move their chair to an inaccessible location. When you transport them to the hospital, be sure to bring their chair with you, make arrangements for someone else to bring it, or if their primary chair is too large or heavy for transport, bring a transport chair or remember to make arrangements at the emergency department (ED) for one to be readily available.

- If they need assistance transferring from the wheelchair to a stair chair or a stretcher, ask them (or family members, if more appropriate) the best way to lift and move them. They make transfer and lift decisions many times a day and can tell you the best and safest way to move the patient.

De-escalation

People with a variety of disabilities can have significant behavioral challenges when faced with an emergency or other experience that is outside their norm. This can be especially true with people with autism, intellectual disabilities, traumatic brain injuries, or mental health concerns. Finding ways to verbally de-escalate a potentially volatile situation without physical or chemical restraint is preferable, not only for the patient but also for the providers as it helps establish rapport, gain trust, and protect the dignity and self-esteem of the agitated/aggressive person.[21]

Agitation is behavior associated with turbulent emotions that may include repetitive behaviors and motor behaviors that are not goal directed, such as foot tapping, rocking, hand flapping, or hair pulling, repetitive thoughts, repetitive vocalizations, irritability, and heightened response to environmental stimuli.[22] Agitation can lead to aggression and violence against self or others and can be compounded by alcohol or substance use.

It is also important to rule out a treatable medical cause for agitation, aggression, and violence, such as the following:[23]

- Alcohol
- Amphetamines
- Cocaine
- Excited delirium (*Note:* This is a medical emergency and should be treated immediately according to local protocols.)
- Stroke
- Head injury
- Hypoglycemia
- Seizures

While law enforcement officers will have had training in verbal de-escalation techniques,[24] it is not something that is covered frequently or in depth in EMS training. Most jurisdictions will have policies in place for EMS to stage off-scene when a patient or family member is believed to be, or is potentially, agitated or violent (this is particularly true for diabetic, psychiatric, and overdose dispatches). This allows law enforcement to clear the scene for EMS to enter safely. However, there are times when either that information is not available at the time of dispatch, it is not believed that there is a behavioral issue on scene, or the individual escalates for medical or psychiatric reasons while providers are on scene.

The first rule of EMS is scene safety. Your safety is paramount as you cannot help others if you are injured. If you are told to stage by dispatch, do so out of view of the scene, and wait for law enforcement to clear the scene for your entry. If you are on scene and the situation deteriorates and you believe your safely is in jeopardy, back out of the scene and request law enforcement backup. This is not the time to be a hero!

Occasionally, a patient is agitated, anxious, or frightened, and they need verbal support and guidance to help them calm themselves, refocus, and allow you to assess, treat, and transport them to the hospital for further evaluation. EMS providers may have a variety of local resources to help with proficiency in de-escalation techniques. Taking a face-to-face course where techniques can be practiced and role-played can be particularly helpful. If those courses are not readily available in your jurisdiction, here are some general suggestions found in the literature.

The big ideas to keep in mind

Richmond et al. describe four broad goals to keep in mind when working with an agitated patient:[25]

1. Ensure the safety of patient and others in the area.

2. Help the patient manage their emotions and maintain/gain control of their behavior.

3. Avoid the use of restraint.

4. Avoid interventions that could escalate the agitation.

The 10 Commandments

In a 2002 article for *Current Psychiatry*, Avrim Fishkind described the "Ten Commandments of De-escalation" (see table 1–3).[26]

1. You shall respect personal space.

- Keep a distance of at least two arms' length between you and the patient, greater if the patient is likely to lash out physically.
- Maintain normal eye contact but do not stare or avert your eyes, which can be interpreted as exhibiting either aggression or fear. Either can exacerbate behavior.
- It is also important to maintain an escape route for both you and the patient. They should not feel trapped or cornered, and you need to be able to leave quickly and safely.

2. You shall not be provocative.

- It is important that you stay verbally and physically calm. Be cautious with your tone of voice; do not have an angry, frustrated, impatient, or irritated tone.
- Keep your body language relaxed. Keep your arms uncrossed, your hands visible, and your fists unclenched (even when arms are hanging down at your sides).
- Do not employ verbal or physical threats.
- Make sure that your tone of voice and body language match.

3. You shall establish verbal contact.

- There may be many people on scene, but only one person should be communicating with the patient. Having multiple people trying to communicate, reason, or convince will be overwhelming and counterproductive.
- Identify yourself by name and position and ask their name.
- Consider the appropriateness of using their first name versus addressing them with their last name. Calling them only by their first name could be perceived as too personal or disrespectful, but using their last name could be viewed as patronizing. When in doubt, ask them how they would like to be addressed.

4. You shall be concise and repeat yourself.

- Fishkind recommends using short words and phrases and simple vocabulary so as not to overwhelm or confuse the patient.[27]
- Due to their agitation, they may not hear you the first (several) times you say something, and they may need additional time to process and understand what you have said.
- Be prepared to repeat yourself, while not showing outwardly in tone or body language any frustration you may be feeling.

5. You shall identify wants and feelings.

- It is important to recognize and acknowledge the patient's needs.
- Be empathetic, state what you are observing, and also offer support. Examples could include, "You seem angry. How can I help?" or "You seem afraid. How can I assure you that you are safe?"

6. You shall listen.

- Listen to what the patient is saying and try not to assign your own interpretations.
- Practice active listening by reflecting back what they are saying using phrases such as, "What I am hearing you say is . . .," "Let me be sure I am understanding what you are saying . . .," or "Tell me if I'm on the right track...."

7. You shall agree or agree to disagree.

- You may not be able to agree with the patient on everything, especially if it involves a delusion or hallucination, but you should be able to find something on which you can agree, even if it is very small. Richmond et al. describe three ways to agree with a patient:[28]
  - *Agree with the truth.* If the patient is upset about the number of law enforcement officers on a scene, you can say, "Yes, there are a lot of officers here tonight."
  - *Agree with the principle.* If the patient claims that his mother stole his belongings, you might say, "I believe people have the right not to have their possessions taken by others."
  - *Agree with the odds.* If the patient is upset because the doctor would not fill their narcotics prescription twice in one week, you can respond with, "I imagine that other people would feel the same way about not being able to fill a prescription."
- At some point, though, you may just have to agree to disagree about a point of contention while acknowledging that the experience or feeling is very real to them.

8. You shall lay down the law.

- It is okay and appropriate to set clear guidelines for what constitutes acceptable behavior and language.
- You will probably be challenged, so be prepared to address that challenge calmly and respectfully.
- It is also appropriate to explain, in a nonthreatening manner, the consequences of their behavior (they could get hurt, restrained, sedated, or arrested) and make it clear that the decision is their choice.

9. You shall offer choices.

 - A patient who is very agitated or feels like there are no options will likely be unable to generate choices, so it is not a good idea to ask them to think of an alternative behavior or action.
 - It can be helpful for you to offer choices that are realistic and possible, such as, "Would you like to discuss this in the kitchen or the living room?" or "I'd like to check your blood sugar. Would you prefer to do that in the ambulance or sitting on the bench?"
 - Never promise something you are not completely sure can be provided. If you give the patient the choice of a soda or a cup of coffee after they put their clothes back on, and there is no coffee, your credibility will suffer.

10. You shall debrief the patient and staff.

 - If de-escalation strategies do not work and the patient ends up physically or chemically restrained, it is appropriate for the person who ordered the restraint to talk to the patient after the crisis has resolved and the patient is calm in order to restore the therapeutic relationship.
 - This final step is often not practical, realistic, or possible for pre-hospital EMS staff who may have no contact with the patient once their care is turned over to hospital staff.
 - It is appropriate, however, for the EMS provider in charge to debrief with the ambulance crew if a patient has had to be chemically or physically restrained. This is an opportunity not only to make sure everyone is physically and emotionally fine (and if not, take the steps necessary to resolve those issues through medical care or critical incident stress management) but also to discuss what went well, what did not go well, and consider suggestions for future events.

Oliva et al. also provide suggestions for behaviors to avoid when dealing with an agitated patient.[29] They recommend the following:

 • Not asking "why" questions as they can make the patient feel defensive about their previous decisions or behaviors. Avoid asking questions such as the following:
   - "Why are you acting like this?"
   - "Why did you take those pills?"
   - "Why didn't you go see your doctor?"

- Not rushing or pressuring the patient to answer a question or make a decision.
  - You may be spending extra time on scene, but you will likely save time in the long run by being able to transport and turn over a calmer, more coherent patient.
- Not taking words or actions personally.
  - It's not about you, even if it feels like it!
- Not allowing personal feelings or experiences to interfere with or otherwise impact words or behaviors.
  - You may have been in a similar situation before, or had a friend or family member experience a mental health crisis, but this is typically not the time to share that experience or make suggestions based on that experience. Stay in the moment and recognize that what worked in one situation may not be appropriate in another.
- Not denying a patient's hallucinations or delusions but also not agreeing that they are real.
  - You can acknowledge that you believe that they are seeing/hearing something that you do not.
  - You can recognize and value their fear or distress about what they are hearing or seeing.
  - It is important to realize that what they are hearing or seeing *is real to them at that time.*

In summary, people with disabilities can potentially present a variety of medical and behavioral challenges for EMS providers, but remember that they are patients, first and foremost. Treat them with compassion and respect, as you would with any patient. Ask thoughtful, considerate questions to help guide your assessments and interventions. The following chapters will give you some specific guidance and suggestions for a variety of disabilities you may encounter in the field.

Table 1–3. The 10 commandments of de-escalation

The Ten Commandments of De-escalation	
1	You shall respect personal space.
2	You shall not be provocative.
3	You shall establish verbal contact.
4	You shall be concise and repeat yourself.
5	You shall identify wants and feelings.
6	You shall listen.
7	You shall agree or agree to disagree.
8	You shall lay down the law.
9	You shall offer choices.
10	You shall debrief the patient and staff.

Source: Fishkind, "Calming Agitation with Words, Not Drugs: 10 Commandments for Safety."

Notes

1. Matthew W. Brault, *Americans with Disabilities: 2010—Household Economic Studies* (Washington, DC: US Census Bureau, US Department of Commerce, 2012); US Department of Commerce, US Census Bureau Public Information Office, "Nearly 1 in 5 People Have a Disability in the U.S., Census Bureau Reports," Newsroom, US Census Bureau, July 25, 2012, https://www.census.gov/newsroom/releases/archives/miscellaneous/cb12-134.html.

2. Brault, *Americans with Disabilities*; US Department of Commerce, US Census Bureau, "Nearly 1 in 5 People Have a Disability in the U.S., Census Bureau Reports."

3. Americans with Disabilities Act of 1990, as amended by the ADA Amendments Act of 2008, 42 U.S.C., Ch. 126, § 12101 (2008): (b)(1)–(b)(2), accessible from https://www.ada.gov/pubs/ada.htm.

4. Luk Cannoodt, Charles Mock, and Maurice Bucagu, "Identifying Barriers to Emergency Care Services," *International Journal of Health Planning and Management* 27, no. 2 (2012): E104–E120, https://doi.org/10.1002/hpm.1098.

5. Cannoodt, Mock, and Bucagu, "Identifying Barriers to Emergency Care Services."

6. Stephen P. Gulley, Elizabeth K. Rasch, and Leighton Chan, "The Complex Web of Health: Relationships among Chronic Conditions, Disability, and Health Services," *Public Health Reports* 126, no. 4 (2011): 495–507, https://doi.org/10.1177/003335491112600406.

7. E. Bancroft et al., "Environmental Barriers to Health Care among Persons with Disabilities—Los Angeles County, California, 2002–2003," *Morbidity & Mortality Weekly Report* 55, no. 48 (2006):1,300–1,303, https://doi.org/10.1037/e574662006-002.

8. Bancroft et al., "Environmental Barriers to Health Care."

9. Gloria L. Krahn, Deborah K. Walker, and Rosaly Correa-De-Araujo, "Persons with Disabilities as an Unrecognized Health Disparity Population," *American Journal of Public Health* 105, no. S2 (2015): S198–S206, https://doi.org/10.2105/ajph.2014.302182.

10. Nancy A. Miller et al., "The Relation between Health Insurance and Health Care Disparities among Adults with Disabilities," *American Journal of Public Health* 104, no. 3 (2014): E85–E93, https://doi.org/10.2105/ajph.2013.301478.

11. Elizabeth K. Rasch, Stephen P. Gulley, and Leighton Chan, "Use of Emergency Departments among Working Age Adults with Disabilities: A Problem of Access and Service Needs," *Health Services Research* 48, no. 4 (2013): 1,334–1,358, https://doi.org/10.1111/1475-6773.12025.

12. Rasch, Gulley, and Chan, "Use of Emergency Departments among Working Age Adults with Disabilities."

13. Rasch, Gulley, and Chan, "Use of Emergency Departments among Working Age Adults with Disabilities."

14. Vicki Wilkins, "Communicating Humanness: Attitudes and Language," *Social Advocacy and Systems Change* 3, no. 1 (2012): 38–43.

15. The Arc of the United States, "What Is People First Language?" https://www.thearc.org/who-we-are/media-center/people-first-language.

16. National Association of the Deaf, "Community and Culture: Frequently Asked Questions," https://www.nad.org/resources/american-sign-language/community-and-culture-frequently-asked-questions/.

17. Dana S. Dunn and Erin E. Andrews, "Person-First and Identity-First Language: Developing Psychologists' Cultural Competence Using Disability Language," *American Psychologist* 70, no. 3 (2015): 255–264, https://doi.org/10.1037/a0038636.

18. US Department of Justice, Civil Rights Division, Disability Rights Section, "ADA Requirements: Service Animal," https://www.ada.gov/service_animals_2010.htm.

19. Americans with Disabilities Act of 1990, Title II Regulations, Part 35, "Nondiscrimination on the Basis of Disability in State and Local Government Services" (October 11, 2016): §35.136(i), https://www.ada.gov/regs2010/titleII_2010/titleII_2010_regulations.htm#a35136.

20. Jacquie Brennan and Vinh Nguyen, *Service Animals and Emotional Support Animals* (Houston, TX: Southwest ADA Center, 2014), https://adata.org/sites/adata.org/files/files/Service_Animal_Booklet_2014(2).pdf.

21. Owen Price and John Baker, "Key Components of De-escalation Techniques: A Thematic Synthesis," *International Journal of Mental Health Nursing* 21, no. 4 (2012): 310–319, https://doi.org/10.1111/j.1447-0349.2011.00793.x.

22. Janet S. Richmond et al., "Verbal De-Escalation of the Agitated Patient: Consensus Statement of the American Association for Emergency Psychiatry Project BETA De-escalation Workgroup," *Western Journal of Emergency Medicine* 13, no. 1 (2012): 17–25, https://doi.org/10.5811/westjem.2011.9.6864.

23. Marina Garriga et al., "Assessment and Management of Agitation in Psychiatry: Expert Consensus," *World Journal of Biological Psychiatry* 17, no. 2 (2016): 86–128, https://doi.org/10.3109/15622975.2015.1132007; and Avrim Fishkind, "Calming Agitation with Words, Not Drugs: 10 Commandments for Safety," *Current Psychiatry* 1, no. 4 (2002): 32–39, https://www.mdedge.com/psychiatry/article/66121/calming-agitation-words-not-drugs-10-commandments-safety.

24. Janet R. Oliva, Rhiannon Morgan, and Michael T. Compton, "A Practical Overview of De-Escalation Skills in Law Enforcement: Helping Individuals in Crisis While Reducing Police Liability and Injury," *Journal of Police Crisis Negotiations* 10, nos. 1–2 (2010): 15–29, https://doi.org/10.1080/15332581003785421.

25. Richmond et al., "Verbal De-Escalation of the Agitated Patient."

26. Fishkind, "Calming Agitation with Words, Not Drugs: 10 Commandments for Safety."

27. Fishkind, "Calming Agitation with Words, Not Drugs: 10 Commandments for Safety."

28. Richmond et al., "Verbal De-escalation of the Agitated Patient."

29. Oliva, Morgan, and Compton, "Practical Overview of De-escalation Skills in Law Enforcement."

2

Autism Spectrum Disorders

You are dispatched to a motor vehicle collision between two SUVs. The first arriving ambulance is treating a patient with facial lacerations. You are directed to the driver of the other vehicle, a 23-year-old man, Daniel, who was at fault and does not appear to be seriously injured. He is complaining of mild left shoulder and arm pain from the seat belt, but it appears that he is having difficulty moving his arm, and his injury might actually be more serious than it initially appears.

When you approach Daniel sitting on the curb, he is visibly agitated and rocking back and forth. As you attempt to gain his attention to introduce yourself and begin your assessment, he responds verbally but without looking at you. You place your hand on his right shoulder to help direct his attention to you, and he abruptly jerks back to avoid your touch. When you ask him to tell you what happened, he responds with irritation that it should be quite obvious to you what happened and refuses to answer any more questions, repeating over and over, "My fault, my fault, my fault," as he continues to rock back and forth. Recognizing that David may have an autism spectrum disorder, you take a step back (literally and figuratively) and start asking specific assessment questions, while signaling to your crew and the rescue squad to give you both some space.

What Is an Autism Spectrum Disorder?

Autism spectrum disorder (ASD) is a complex disorder that has become more prevalent in recent decades. Prior to the late 1980s, one rarely saw mention of autism in the mainstream media. Today most people are aware of the existence of autism, even if they are not certain of the specifics of the disorder. In 2000,

93,000 US children received special education services under the category of autism. In 2013, that number rose to 538,000. According to the Centers for Disease Control and Prevention, it is estimated that 1 in 59 children has ASD, with boys four times as likely (1 in 37) to be identified than girls.[1] This is an increase from 1 in 68 children in 2012 data.[2]

While ASD is seen across all races, ethnicities, and cultures, its prevalence is higher in white, non-Hispanic children when compared to black (20% higher), Asian/Pacific islander (40% higher), and Hispanic (50% higher) children.[3] This is believed to be due not to a genuinely higher rate of ASD in white children but to sociocultural factors surrounding identification and diagnosis. Issues such as stigma, immigration status, language barriers, healthcare access, and finances all contribute to minority children being less likely to be identified with ASD.

While it is true that the number of people being identified with ASD has appeared to skyrocket, it is believed that the increase is not due to an "epidemic" of the disorder but from better understanding and recognition of ASD, a push for earlier identification, and reduced stigma.[4]

One alleged cause of autism, vaccines, has been thoroughly disproven. In 1998 a British gastroenterologist named Andrew Wakefield published a paper in the *Lancet* linking the measles, mumps, and rubella (MMR) vaccination to the development of autism. The paper received a lot of publicity, and as a result, vaccine rates dropped, and illness rates increased. In 2010 the paper was retracted by the *Lancet* when it was found that the research was fraudulent due to ethical violations and poor research methods.[5] The original, flawed findings have not been confirmed in additional studies.

ASD can be diagnosed in children by a health care provider (pediatrician, psychologist, psychiatrist, etc.) or by school personnel as part of a special education assessment process. The diagnostic criteria for ASD are identified in the *Diagnostic and Statistical Manual of Mental Disorders* from the American Psychiatric Association and in the World Health Organization's *International Statistical Classification of Diseases and Related Health Problems*.[6]

The primary characteristics of ASD are problems with social interaction and communication; restricted/repetitive interests, behaviors, and language; and hypersensitivity or hyposensitivity, or both, to environmental stimuli. These issues vary in specific manifestations and severity by the individual and by the situation. Some people with ASD might be nearly indistinguishable from "neurotypical" people, appearing only immature, shy, and/or "slightly nerdy." But when the individuals are in a stressful medical or traumatic emergency situation, ASD characteristics can "flare up" and have a significant impact on behavior and communication. Others with ASD are more impacted on a daily basis. Some may not speak or have difficulty with communication; have significant interfering behaviors like rituals, rocking, hand flapping, and saying the same thing over and over; and have self-injurious behaviors such as head banging or skin picking. People with ASD are also more likely to need care at the emergency department due to psychiatric issues, aggressive behavior, self-harming behaviors, and seizures.[7]

Social Interaction and Communication Deficits

Eye contact

People with ASD can have difficulty with social interaction and using language in social situations. A common characteristic of people with ASD is having limited eye contact, which is an important component of communication. Think about how much information can be gained from a social interaction if you are able to look at the person you are conversing with. Eye contact helps a person attend to the conversation. Seeing the faces of the people you are talking with allows you to infer mood, frame of mind, and communicative intent.

Poor eye contact can manifest as being completely unable to look a person in the eye (e.g., by looking at the floor, the neck, or over the shoulder of the conversation partner) or by glancing away frequently. Be aware, however, that in many cultures direct eye contact is considered rude, especially to a person in authority (e.g., some Asian, Native American, and Hispanic cultures) and does not imply a patient has ASD. This can be frustrating for the person on the receiving end of the poor eye contact, as they may not know if the patient is paying attention or listening to them. It can feel disconcerting at best, and at worst, disrespectful. And while it may feel as if the person is not paying attention, they may in fact be attempting to pay better attention.

Some people with ASD find maintaining eye contact causes stress and anxiety, even to the point of becoming physically uncomfortable.[8] Other people on the spectrum have described difficulty paying attention to both a person's face *and* their words. Many people with ASD misinterpret or do not understand facial expressions and/or body language. As a result, visual input distracts them from the verbal input, so they reduce the visual input in order to more fully attend to the verbal. For others, the process of trying to decide what is socially appropriate eye contact is uncomfortable and confusing, and the verbal input is lost while concentrating on how to negotiate the eye contact. Consequently they attempt to minimize the visual input.

Whatever the reason, this can have an impact on EMS assessment of an individual with ASD as we attempt to gain the trust of our patient. If they do not look at us, it can be difficult to establish the trust that runs both ways in a patient-provider relationship. It may feel like our patient is not being honest and forthright with us when they do not look at us when answering questions. Knowing that reduced eye contact is not due to deception but rather discomfort or an attempt to better process verbal input can help to alleviate concerns about whether your patient is answering questions honestly.

Language

Verbal and nonverbal language issues are ubiquitous in people with ASD. By definition and diagnostic criteria, people with ASD will demonstrate difficulties with verbal and nonverbal language. It may be delayed, have unusual usage, or may be absent altogether. Some individuals with ASD have no delays in their language acquisition (and may even be highly verbal) but are awkward in their language usage, having difficulty with pragmatic language, or the social component of language. Three linguistic categories where difficulties are seen with individuals with ASD are semantics, syntax, and pragmatics.

Semantics. *Semantics* are the rules surrounding word meaning and correct word usage.[9] People with ASD can have unusual semantic issues with language. Children often have difficulty with the accurate labeling of items, sometimes using *neologisms*, or made up words. Children may identify items with a more general term in the same category ("animal" instead of "dog") or a more specific one (calling all animals "dog"). They may use another word in the same category ("truck" instead of "car"). Or they may use a vague description instead of the name ("sweet drink" for "soda").[10] It can complicate an EMS assessment if you ask your patient to identify the location of their pain and they say "arm" when they may mean they have pain in their hand (underspecification) or their leg (incorrect label in the same category). You may focus your assessment on the wrong area.

Syntax. *Syntax* refers to how words are put together to make sentences, including the rules of grammar.[11] A common syntactic error in children with ASD is pronoun reversal, such as substituting "you" or "we" for "me." This is likely due to concurrent issues with pragmatic language and echolalia (see more on echolalia below).[12] Instead of responding to the question "Do you have any pain?" with "I have a headache," the patient may respond, "You have a headache."

Pragmatics. *Pragmatic language* encompasses not only the words we say but also how we say them, why we say them, and the context in which we say them, as well as our body language and tone of voice. The American Speech-Language-Hearing Association identifies three pragmatic language skills:[13]

1. Using language for different purposes (and choosing the correct purpose), such as greeting, informing, demanding, promising, and requesting

2. Changing language to meet the specific needs of a situation, such as speaking with a child versus an adult, talking with a parent versus a police officer, or communicating urgency in an emergency

3. Following cultural rules for conversations, such as turn taking, staying on topic, recognizing when someone has lost interest, when and how to interrupt, and ending a conversation

Pragmatic challenges may make those with ASDs appear rude, disinterested, or aloof, especially when coupled with poor eye contact. They may have a tone of voice that is singsong or flat and robotic. Many may not know how to start or end a conversation gracefully. They may dominate the conversation about a single subject, interrupt without understanding the back and forth of a conversation, and/or abruptly walk away from a conversation. People with ASDs also have trouble reading body language and facial expressions and may not understand tone of voice, including sarcasm. Everyone has times when they do not understand their role in a conversation or misunderstand something that was said and subsequently respond inappropriately. However, people with ASD have pragmatic issues that persist past an age-appropriate level, manifest across all social settings, and increase during periods of stress or anxiety.

In addition, there can be difficulty with figurative language. If you use idiomatic phrases, your patient may be confused. Consider the literal meanings of these questions, all of which may be asked as part of an EMS assessment:

- Are you feeling a bit under the weather?
- Do you have butterflies in your stomach?
- Any problems with your sugar?

While most people understand that these questions refer to feeling unwell, having an unsettled/upset stomach, and having unstable blood glucose levels, respectively, a person with ASD may be unsure how to answer. In their minds, they are obviously above ground, have not swallowed any insects, and do not drink sweetened tea. Being literal in phrasing questions or statements if you know or suspect an ASD can help facilitate clear communication.

While problems with semantics, syntax, and pragmatics may not have a significant negative impact on an EMS assessment and subsequent treatment, they can cause a breakdown in communication and increased confusion with subsequent frustration on the parts of both provider and patient. Echolalia, however, has the potential to have a significant negative impact on the provider-patient relationship.

Echolalia

Echolalia is the repetition of another person's words, phrases, or sentences[14] that may *appear* to be meaningless or noncommunicative but actually does serve communicative purposes. Simply speaking, echolalia is when the person with whom you are speaking repeats back to you something you have said or something they have heard previously. The purpose of echolalic utterances may be unclear, even in context, but Stiegler notes that echolalia can serve a variety of purposes, including practice/rehearsal of language, labeling, requesting, directing, acknowledging, and answering,[15] as well as an attempt to self-regulate behavior.[16]

Echolalia can be delayed or immediate. With *delayed echolalia*, which is defined as occurring at least two conversational turns away from the original utterance,[17] the individual may repeat television or movie dialogue, sing parts of songs, recite text from books, and so on. This delayed repetition can be minutes, hours, days, weeks, or months after they first heard the words. Delayed echolalia can appear to be nonpurposeful, especially when the repeated words are significantly out of context from the current situation. For example, a person with ASD being assessed during an emergency situation may repeat over and over, "The TV is broken. The TV is broken," and this sentence appears to be completely unrelated to the current situation. For the individual, however, they may be using language that evokes another time when they were very upset (when their television was not working). While it may seem out of context, for the person with ASD, it is relevant.

Immediate echolalia will occur immediately after the original comment and can consist of all or part of the utterance. Immediate echolalia can present challenges to an EMS assessment, and providers will want to ask their questions carefully. Consider the question, "Do you have chest pain or a headache?" A person who displays immediate echolalia with only part of the utterance may respond, "Headache." It may be impossible to know if the response is an accurate answer to the question or if the individual is actually saying that they have chest pain, both headache and chest pain, or neither. Additionally, the repetition of the question by the person with ASD may appear to indicate that they don't understand the question, causing the EMS provider to repeat or rephrase the question, and potentially confusing, frustrating, or upsetting the patient.

While it might be impossible for the listener, especially one unfamiliar with the specific language characteristics of the patient, to be able to discern the purpose of the patient's echolalic utterances, simply being aware of the potential complexities to assessment and treatment when echolalia is present can help limit and/or mitigate potential errors.

Theory of mind

A hallmark of ASD is having deficits in *theory of mind*, which is the understanding that people have different interpretations of experiences, even shared experiences. People who have a strong theory of mind are able to recognize that other people have thoughts, feelings, and experiences that are different from their own, even when they have shared the same or similar experiences, events, or conversations.[18] People with theory of mind deficits, however, struggle with understanding that people can have different experiences and different understandings of experiences. This can lead to confusion and breakdowns in communication. In social situations, this can result in one-sided conversations because those with ASD may assume that everyone is as interested in science fiction or roller coasters as they are. It also can create confusion when those with ASD do not communicate their expectations for social plans because if they know the date, time, and location for meeting up, their friends must know as well. This can be more serious in a prehospital emergency setting.

For example, a person with ASD is being assessed for generalized sickness and has abdominal pain. He knows he has abdominal pain, but due to theory of mind deficits he assumes that you *also* know he has abdominal pain and so does not tell you. If you do not do a complete and thorough assessment, this important symptom may go unrecorded because your patient assumes that you know what he knows about his pain. But let's assume you have done a complete SAMPLE and OPQRST assessment and ask your patient about pain. (*Note:* SAMPLE—signs/symptoms, allergies, medications, pertinent medical history, last oral intake, events leading to the illness/injury; OPQRST—onset, provocation of pain/illness, quality of pain/illness, radiation of pain, severity of symptoms, time since onset.) He then might respond with frustration and irritation because he expects that you should already be aware of that symptom. And because of the previously mentioned challenges with the use of language, the patient may also have difficulty describing and quantifying his pain.

Restricted/repetitive behaviors and language

People with ASD frequently exhibit physical behaviors and language that can appear odd or unusual or may be disruptive. These behaviors can take different forms, including perseverative or persistent behaviors and self-stimulatory behaviors.

For some people with ASD, perseverative behaviors, including perseverative language, can be self-stimulatory in nature and are rhythmic and repetitive (discussed in more detail below). For others, perseverative behaviors manifest as topic or content persistence[19] where the individual fixates on a topic (sports, airplanes, US presidents, etc.) without regard for the interest or inclusion of their conversational partner, or relentless questioning that has communicative intent and persists even after their question has been answered.[20] While harmless, this persistent verbal discourse can be boring or irritating to others, leading them to limit social interactions with the person with ASD. These verbal behaviors can become more prevalent during times of stress or anxiety.

Self-stimulatory behaviors

Self-stimulatory behaviors, or motor and verbal stereotypical behaviors (sometimes informally called "stimming"), are common with people with ASD and are seen in up to 70% of diagnosed individuals.[21] The stereotypic behavior is rhythmic and repetitive, appears to be nonfunctional, and can appear for a myriad of reasons such as anxiety, sensory over- or understimulation, stress, boredom, happiness, and excitement. These behaviors may seem like they serve no purpose, but for the individual the behaviors can be calming or soothing, or serve as a way to gain needed sensory input.[22] Goldman et al. describe a wide range of behaviors including facial grimacing; lip, tongue, and mouth movements; full body rocking/spinning; hand flapping, waving, and clapping; hair pulling/twirling; and many others.[23]

Stereotypic/self-stimulatory behavior, by definition, is not dangerous and does not need to be stopped. However, some individuals exhibit stereotypic behaviors that are self-injurious and harmful, such as head-banging, skin picking, or slapping themselves. When these behaviors are present, the person should be gently redirected to a more appropriate behavior that serves the same purpose as the harmful behavior. For example, if the person is biting themselves due to anxiety, giving them something else to bite on may alleviate the harmful behavior.

When a person with ASD is experiencing a medical or traumatic emergency, their stereotypic behavior can increase and become more interfering, potentially having a negative impact on your assessment and subsequent treatment. Taking a blood pressure, conducting a 12-lead EKG, or measuring a blood glucose level can all be difficult if frequent, repetitive body movements are present. It can also be difficult to direct their attention to your necessary assessment questions. While these behaviors are not inherently dangerous, this would be another time where it would be appropriate to *temporarily* redirect the behaviors with something less interfering, like giving someone who is hand flapping something to hold and squeeze in their hands. This is not intended to permanently eliminate or stop the behavior, but simply to attempt to allow you to conduct the pieces of your assessment that you are unable to obtain due to the behaviors.

Hypersensitivity and/or hyposensitivity to environmental stimuli

People with ASD can have unusual responses to environmental stimuli. They can be over- or hypersensitive, under- or hyposensitive, or they may crave or seek out intense sensory experiences. This difficulty with processing environmental stimuli can also be called sensory processing disorder. In a groundbreaking book, *The Out-Of-Sync Child: Recognizing and Coping with Sensory Processing Disorder*, Carol S. Kranowitz defines *sensory processing disorder* as "the inability to use information received through the senses in order to function smoothly in daily life."[24] People without ASD can have sensory processing disorder, but as many as 95% of people with ASD will have some difficulty with sensory processing.[25] This can lead to behavior issues as the individuals attempt to avoid unpleasant sensory input or seek out input they are craving.[26]

Sensory processing problems can occur within the five well-known senses of vision, hearing (auditory), smell, taste, and touch (tactile), but they can also occur with the less familiar senses of vestibular and proprioception. The *vestibular sense*, located in the semicircular canals of the inner ear, is our sense of balance and spatial orientation, allowing us to coordinate movement with balance. The *proprioceptive sense* is the awareness of body orientation in space and of the force needed by muscles for various tasks.[27] For example, without being consciously aware of it, people use a different level of force to put an arm through the sleeve of a lightweight summer blouse than they do for a heavy winter coat. Have you ever picked up a glass of water, thinking it was heavier than it was, and spilled the contents because you picked it up with too much force? That's a function of your proprioceptive sense.

When people have a hypersensitivity to a sensory input, they cannot modulate, regulate, or inhibit the input that they are receiving. For these individuals, the response to this uninhibited sensory input can range from irritation, to feeling overwhelmed, to outright fear, and they respond accordingly. Some may respond with irritation and frustration, but others may respond with avoidance, crying, fear, or even aggressive behaviors as they try to reduce the sensory input that is causing physical and emotional distress.

Consider a scenario with a 10-year-old child with ASD who does not communicate verbally and has a hypersensitivity to flashing lights. You are at the scene of a motor vehicle collision in the late evening, and the emergency lights are flashing. The lights are especially bright and visible due to the time of day. Your patient is not badly injured, but he needs an assessment on scene and transport to the emergency department for some sutures for a small laceration. Being around flashing lights causes disorientation and pain, but your patient is unable to use verbal language to let the people around him know that the lights hurt. What is a natural response for him? To remove or reduce the painful/ unpleasant stimulus. This child has a variety of ways to do this. He can remove himself from the lights by running away, or he can hide his face inside his hoodie and put his head down. He can try to stop the lights by attempting to get into the ambulance cab to flip the light switch, or he might kick and scream at you, trying to get you to turn the lights off. Remember that since he cannot communicate verbally, you will not know what he is asking. He might even try throwing something at the light bar on the ambulance. As an EMS provider, you might not realize the root cause of the behavior (painful sensory stimulus) and only see the behavioral result (aggressive, destructive, or withdrawn behavior). If you respond to the behavior as presented, consider a typical course of action:

- If he runs away, you've lost your patient.
- If he hides inside his hoodie and covers his face, you might be tempted to do what would generally be appropriate with a neurotypical individual. You would go up to him, maybe put a gentle hand on his arm, and pull the hoodie down to see his face. In the person with ASD and sensory processing disorder, however, this could cause more anxiety and distress as the unfamiliar sensory input will be increased.
- If he tries to get into the ambulance cab, assaults you, or attempts to damage the ambulance, law enforcement will likely become involved, which could include raised voices, increased touching, and possible restraint.

While you may not be able to predict or prevent these scenarios from happening (especially if you are late on scene or do not know the individual has ASD), approaching a situation with the idea that what appears to be inappropriate or aggressive behavior might actually be rooted in a physical cause can help you consider alternative interactions and approaches with your out-of-control patient. This way you can act as their advocate rather than their adversary, which is easy to do when behaviors are scary.

Table 2–1 outlines some possible characteristics of people with hyposensitivity or hypersensitivity to the seven senses. Not all people with ASD will exhibit all of these characteristics. As you read through the list, think about how these characteristics can be impacted by an emergency situation.

Table 2–1. Possible characteristics of hyposensitivity and hypersensitivity relating to the senses

	Possible Characteristics of Hyposensitivity and Hypersensitivity Relating to the Senses		
Sense	**Hyposensitive** (not as sensitive to stimuli)	**Hypersensitive** (oversensitive to stimuli)	**Seeking/craving** (wants more stimuli)
Auditory	• Appears not to hear sounds or voices • Appears unaware of sounds in the environment	• Actively avoids sounds (hides, covers ears, wears headphones without device attached) • Appears anxious or frightened by sounds (emergency sirens, frequent, rapid questioning by EMS providers)	• Enjoys noisy places • Increases the volume on the television • Creates his/her own noise
Visual	• Does not pay attention to visual input (traffic lights, street signs, written directions) • Stares at people or objects without apparent recognition • Does not respond quickly to visual stimulus	• Avoids visual input, especially from bright or flickering lights (emergency response lights, ambulance cabin lights) • Wears sunglasses, even at night • Has trouble negotiating rapidly moving objects like walking around people, a swing, or a thrown ball	• Stares at flickering lights or sunlight • Spends a lot of time looking at a screen (television, computer, tablet)

Table 2–1. . . . *continued*

Taste	• Eats nonfood items (dirt, glue, paper) • Prefers strongly flavored foods (spicy, sour, hot) • Chews clothes, fingers, hair	• Avoids certain food textures (chewy, crunchy, soft) • Avoids certain food flavors or eats very bland foods • Gags or vomits when eating • Has a very limited diet	• Seeks out certain food textures (chewy, crunchy, soft) • Eats nonfood items
Smell	• Unaware of unpleasant or dangerous odors • Eats inappropriate things because of not noticing unpleasant or bad smells	• Easily overwhelmed by odors in the environment • Refuses to eat foods due to their smell • Feels or becomes ill due to household chemical smells	• Enjoys and seeks out certain smells (candles, perfume, fragrance sprays) • Excessively smells clothing, toys, food, people
Tactile	• Does not recognize physical touch, even if it is painful or uncomfortable • Does not recognize when face or hands are dirty • May underreact to pain	• Reacts strongly to touch, even gentle touch (but enjoys or seeks out deep pressure touch) • Is apprehensive or afraid of anticipated touch • Reacts very strongly (out of proportion to the injury) to painful stimuli	• Touches everything (objects and people) • Often bumps into things, rolls or lies on the floor • Craves deep physical pressure and contact with skin

Table 2–1. ...*continued*

Vestibular	• May not be physically active • Does not recognize the sensation of falling so does not respond to protect from possible injury	• Feels insecure while standing, walking, or running • Feels ill with ordinary movement (riding in a car or on a bicycle, playground games, etc.)	• Seeks gross motor movement (running, jumping, spinning, falling, swinging, climbing) • Exhibits impulsive physical behaviors or appears to be a thrill seeker
Proprio-ception	• Appears clumsy and unaware of his/her body • Often bumps into things, drops things, or injures self • Has low muscle tone	• Appears tense, stiff, uncoordinated • Resists/avoids movement, especially those that are weight-bearing • May be a picky eater	• Bumps and falls into walls, floors, furniture, and people • Stomps feet • May wear tight clothes or shoes and/or like to be swaddled past infancy • Chews on nonfood items and likes crunchy/chewy foods

Source: Adapted from Carol S. Kranowitz, *The Out-Of-Sync Child: Recognizing and Coping with Sensory Processing Disorder* (New York: Perigee, 2006).

Of particular concern for EMS providers is the patient who underresponds to pain since this can seriously impact a medical or trauma assessment. Yasuda et al. in their study reported that people with ASD demonstrated a hyposensitivity to pain and had different emotional responses to pain compared to the control group.[28] EMS providers assessing individuals with ASD for pain will want to be aware that their patients may report minimal pain when in fact they may have a significant injury or illness. A reported absence of pain should be considered within that context. Also, individuals who seek certain flavors or textures to satisfy the need for increased oral sensory input may eat substances that are dangerous, poisonous, or not intended to be eaten. Accidental poisoning should be considered in your differential diagnosis when assessing patients.

Seizures

Children with ASD have an increased risk of seizures. Research indicates that seizures occur in 12% to 26% (or possibly more) of children with ASD, compared to about 1% of the general US population.[29] The prevalence of seizures is increased in children who have autism *and* an intellectual disability when compared to those with autism but no intellectual disability. Those with more significant intellectual/cognitive impairments are at greater risk than those with milder intellectual impairments.[30] Emergency department visits due to seizures for children with ASD are estimated to be 14 times greater than seizure-related visits for children without ASD.[31]

Wandering/Elopement

You may be called to help search for or care for a person with ASD who has wandered or *eloped* (run away) from home, school, or family when out in public. Wandering and elopement are common in children with ASD. As many as one-third to one-half of children with ASD, both with and without an intellectual disability (see chapter 3), have been reported to have wandered away or become lost from their caregivers.[32] They may wander to avoid something unpleasant, because they see something they want, or because they are seeking or avoiding sensory stimulation.

Wandering can happen even with close supervision. Recall that individuals with ASD often have challenges with theory of mind and knowing that their understanding of a situation is not the same as that of the people with them. Imagine a child at the store with his parents who decides he wants to look at the toy aisle. He has a clear understanding of what he wants to do and where he wants to go and assumes that his parents also know that he has this desire. So he walks over to the toy aisle without telling his parents. He assumes they share his understanding. Similar wandering can happen in any of the following situations, to name a few:

- The noise is too loud at the amusement park, and he tries to find a place to avoid the noise.

- He tries to avoid the math assignment that has just been given in the classroom, so he bolts out of the building.
- Something new and interesting at the park catches his eye, so he runs toward it.
- He has a fascination with bridges, so he decides to go looking for some to cross.

There are a multitude of other reasons why a child might wander from his parents or caregiver.

A survey of more than 400 parents asked them to identify the possible reasons why their children wandered or eloped.[33] The parents believed the top five reasons behind their child's wandering to be the following:

- Enjoys running/exploring
- Is trying to reach a preferred place
  (e.g., park, playground, home, etc.)
- Is trying to avoid/escape an unpreferred place
  (e.g., school, store, etc.)
- Is pursuing a special interest
  (e.g., looking for bridges, cars, airplanes, etc.)
- Is trying to avoid unpleasant sensory/environmental stimuli
  (e.g., noises, smells, etc.)

When asked about their understanding of their child's state of mind when they wandered, most of the parents said they believed their child was happy and purposeful rather than anxious, sad, or confused.[34]

There are obvious risks to people with ASD who have become separated from their caregivers, depending on the time of day/year they are lost, the ambient temperature, additional risks for injury, and so on. People with ASD may have an inherent attraction to water (it can be calming, as well as visually and auditorily interesting), which has obvious dangers. Drowning has been reported as the leading cause of wandering/elopement deaths for people with ASD.[35] People with ASD who have wandered are at increased risk for abduction, assault, and hypothermia or hyperthermia; injury from animals, falling, or traffic; drowning; sunburn; hunger; or dehydration. These individuals may also hide from their caregivers and those who are trying to locate them, extending their time away. Difficulty with language or lack of verbal communication can contribute to a negative outcome.

If you are called to help with searching for a lost person with ASD, you should, of course, follow the guidelines and search parameters of the scene commander, but someone will want to be sure to communicate with the missing individual's parents or caregivers to find out if there are things to do or avoid. A person who is terrified of dogs is likely to hide from search and rescue dogs. If the person does not respond to their name being called and is hypersensitive to loud voices, shouting their name over and over may not have any positive effect. But if they respond positively to singing and are eager to participate in singing activities, singing their favorite songs may be more effective. Be sure to ask the parents/caregivers about suggestions for successful interactions once the person is located. Will they respond to food? To humor? What are their special interests that could help start a discussion and facilitate rapport?

The National Autism Society provides suggestions for how to interact with the person with ASD once they have been located:[36]

- Remain calm, even though you are excited to find them.
- Limit opportunities to flee again but do not actively restrain them unless they are in imminent danger.
- Reunite them with their parents/caregivers as soon as possible.
- Be prepared to treat injury or illness.
- Remember to be careful about sensory issues and avoid unnecessary touch or noises.
- Use information gained from family members about the person to help make connections. For example, if you know that their favorite show is coming on television very soon, you can start a conversation about the show and encourage them to come with you so they can watch the show.

Implications for EMS

Note: For patients with ASD and an intellectual disability, be sure to review the suggestions in chapter 3, "Intellectual Disabilities."

Implications for EMS staff include the following:

- **Move slowly while explaining what you are going to do before you do it.** Of course, this might be limited by the severity of the situation, but if you consider the old adage "Haste makes waste," sometimes taking a little bit of extra time at the beginning to do something right will save time in the long run. When working with someone with ASD, peppering them with assessment questions and touching them without sufficient explanation may cause them to become anxious and resistant, causing the entire process to take longer.

- **Don't expect or try to force eye contact.** Consider sitting to your patient's side rather than in front of them when asking questions. This can help to reduce the expectation of eye contact and limit visual input.

- **Conduct exams distal to proximal when possible** as you work to gain your patient's trust.

- **Limit physical contact as much as possible.** It is natural for EMS providers to want to lay a reassuring hand on their patient's shoulder or offer to hold their hand. As noted in table 2–1, it is not uncommon for gentle touch to feel painful or threatening to people with hypersensitivity to touch. Ask before you touch and explain why you need to touch.

- **Do not assume negative or aggressive behaviors are rooted in psychiatric issues.** Aggressive or self-harming behavior can occur in response to pain or from hypersensitivity to auditory, visual, or other environmental stimuli. It can also be the result of communication deficits or from generally being overwhelmed by the situation. Discover and mitigate things that could be causing inappropriate behavior.

- **Assume cognitive competence, even if the patient does not communicate with their voice.** Verbal ability with ASDs does not necessarily correlate with cognitive ability. Until you learn otherwise, speak to the patient as you would to anyone else the same age, and adjust as appropriate. Some people with ASDs who are typically verbal communicators can have increased challenges with talking when faced with an emergency situation.

- **Use concrete language (avoid figurative language).** Try to avoid using idioms (sick as a dog, pale as a ghost) that could potentially confuse your patient.

- **Ask specific questions.** Such questions could include, "Does anything hurt?" or "Why did you call 911 today?" rather than, "What's going on today?"

- **Be prepared for echolalia.** Ask questions in multiple ways to reduce potential confusion. If you ask, "Do you have pain in your belly or head?" you might get the response "head" or "belly or head." You might try asking them to show you where it hurts, or to write it down.

- **Check for understanding.** This must be undertaken while still being cautious not to appear that you are talking down to them.

- **Be prepared for bolting or refusal.** The stress and anxiety created by an emergency situation can cause a flight response. It can also cause the individual with ASD to "shut down" and refuse care or to stop responding to you.

- **Allow a familiar face during transport.** If your company does not allow family members in the patient compartment, having a familiar person in the passenger seat may help to alleviate your patient's concerns and allow for that person to be quickly accessible during transport and at the hospital.

- **Reduce sensory stimulation.** Consider the following:
  - Dimming ambulance cabin lights.
  - Not using emergency lights and sirens.
  - Limiting unnecessary EMS personnel in the ambulance.
  - Avoid unnecessary assessments and interventions. This is not the time to let the student insert an IV because they need the practice or to put the patient on the 3-lead because "we do that for everyone" if it is not currently medically necessary.

- **Explain what will happen.** The explanation should include what will happen during transport as well as after arriving at the hospital.

- **Notify hospital personnel of the autism spectrum disorder diagnosis on arrival.** Be prepared for longer turnover, and be your patient's advocate. Let the ER staff know what was successful for you in establishing rapport with your patient so they do not have to figure it out for themselves and potentially delay care further.

Notes

1. Jon Baio et al., "Prevalence of Autism Spectrum Disorder among Children Aged 8 Years—Autism and Developmental Disabilities Monitoring Network, 11 Sites, United States, 2014," *Morbidity and Mortality Weekly Report Summaries* 67, no. 6 (2018): 1–23, https://doi.org/10.15585/mmwr.ss6706a1.

2. Deborah L. Christensen et al., "Prevalence and Characteristics of Autism Spectrum Disorder among Children Aged 8 Years—Autism and Developmental Disabilities Monitoring Network, 11 Sites, United States," *Surveillance Summaries* 65, no. 3 (2016): 1–23, http://dx.doi.org/10.15585/mmwr.ss6503a1.

3. Christiansen et al., "Prevalence and Characteristics of ASD among Children Aged 8 Years."

4. Roy R. Grinker, *Unstrange Minds: Remapping the World of Autism* (Philadelphia: Basic Books, 2007).

5. "Retraction—Ileal-Lymphoid-Nodular Hyperplasia, Non-Specific Colitis, and Pervasive Developmental Disorder in Children," *Lancet* 375, no. 9,713 (2010): 445, https://doi.org/10.1016/s0140-6736(10)60175-4; Fiona Godlee, Jane Smith, and Harvey Marcovitch, "Wakefield's Article Linking MMR Vaccine and Autism Was Fraudulent," *BMJ* 342, no. 7,788 (2011): 64–66, https://doi.org/10.1136/bmj.c7452; and Laura Eggertson, "Lancet Retracts 12-Year-Old Article Linking Autism to MMR Vaccines," *Canadian Medical Association Journal* 182, no. 4 (2010): E199–E200, https://doi.org/10.1503/cmaj.109-3179.

6. American Psychiatric Association, *Diagnostic and Statistical Manual of Mental Disorders*, 5th ed., DSM-5 (Washington, DC: American Psychiatric Association, 2013); and World Health Organization, *International Statistical Classification of Diseases and Related Health Problems*, 10th ed., ICD-10 (Geneva: World Health Organization, 1992), https://apps.who.int/iris/bitstream/handle/10665/37958/9241544228_eng.pdf?sequence=8&isAllowed=y.

7. Dorothea A. Iannuzzi et al., "Brief Report: Emergency Department Utilization by Individuals with Autism," *Journal of Autism and Developmental Disorders* 45, no. 4 (2015): 1,096–1,102, https://doi.org/10.1007/s10803-014-2251-2.

8. Nouchine Hadjikhani et al., "Look Me in the Eyes: Constraining Gaze in the Eye-Region Provokes Abnormally High Subcortical Activation in Autism," *Scientific Reports* 7, no. 3,163 (2017): 1–7, https://doi.org/10.1038/s41598-017-03378-5.

9. Krista M. Wilkinson, "Profiles of Language and Communication Skills in Autism," *Mental Retardation and Developmental Disabilities Research Reviews, Special Issue: Autism* 4, no. 2 (1998): 73–79, https://doi.org/10.1002/(SICI)1098-2779(1998)4:2<73::AID-MRDD3>3.0.CO;2-Y.

10. Wilkinson, "Profiles of Language and Communication Skills in Autism"; and I. Vogindroukas, V. Papageorgiou, and P. Vostanis, "Pattern of Semantic Errors in Autism," *Autism* 7, no. 2 (2003): 195–203, https://doi.org/10.1177/1362361303007002006.

11. Wilkinson, "Profiles of Language and Communication Skills in Autism."

12. Wilkinson, "Profiles of Language and Communication Skills in Autism."

13. American Speech-Language-Hearing Association, "Social Communication," https://www.asha.org/public/speech/development/Social-Communication/.

14. Marina Mergl and Cíntia Alvez Salgado Azoni, "Echolalia's Types in Children with Autism Spectrum Disorder," *Revista CEFAC* 17, no. 6 (2015): 2,072–2,080; and Lillian N. Stiegler, "Examining the Echolalia Literature: Where Do Speech-Language Pathologists Stand?" *American Journal of Speech-Language Pathology* 24, no. 4 (2015): 750–762, https://doi.org/10.1044/2015_ajslp-14-0166.

15. Stiegler, "Examining the Echolalia Literature."

16. Barry M. Prizant and Patrick J. Rydell, "Analysis of Functions of Delayed Echolalia in Autistic Children," *Journal of Speech, Language, and Hearing Research* 27, no. 2 (1984): 183–192, https://doi.org/10.1044/jshr.2702.183.

17. Stiegler, "Examining the Echolalia Literature."

18. Livia Colle, Simon Baron-Cohen, and Jacqueline Hill, "Do Children with Autism Have a Theory of Mind? A Non-Verbal Test of Autism vs. Specific Language Impairment," *Journal of Autism and Developmental Disorders* 37, no. 4 (2007): 716–723, https://doi.org/10.1007/s10803-006-0198-7; and Elif Gökçen, Norah Frederickson, and K. V. Petrides, "Theory of Mind and Executive Control Deficits in Typically Developing Adults and Adolescents with High Levels of Autism Traits," *Journal of Autism and Developmental Disorders*, 46, no. 6 (2016): 2,072–2,087, https://doi.org/10.1007/s10803-016-2735-3.

19. T. Arora, "Understanding the Perseveration Displayed by Students with Autism Spectrum Disorder," *Education* 132, no. 4 (2012): 799–808.

20. Stiegler, "Examining the Echolalia Literature."

21. S. Goldman et al., "Motor Stereotypies in Children with Autism and Other Developmental Disorders," *Developmental Medicine & Child Neurology* 51, no. 1 (2009): 30–38, https://doi.org/10.1111/j.1469-8749.2008.03178.x.

22. Allison B. Cunningham and Laura Schreibman, "Stereotypy in Autism: The Importance of Function," *Research in Autism Spectrum Disorders* 2, no. 3 (2008): 469–479, https://doi.org/10.1016/j.rasd.2007.09.006; and Nicole M. Mays, Jennifer Beal-Alvarez, and Kristine Jolivette, "Using Movement-Based Sensory Interventions to Address Self-Stimulatory Behaviors in Students with Autism," *TEACHING Exceptional Children* 43, no. 6 (2011): 46–52, https://doi.org/10.1177/004005991104300605.

23. Goldman et al., "Motor Stereotypies in Children with Autism."

24. Carol S. Kranowitz, *The Out-Of-Sync Child: Recognizing and Coping with Sensory Processing Disorder* (New York: Perigee, 2006), 9.

25. Yuka Yasuda et al., "Sensory Cognitive Abnormalities of Pain in Autism Spectrum Disorder: A Case Control Study," *Annals of General Psychiatry* 15, no. 8 (2016): 1–8, https://doi.org/10.1186/s12991-016-0095-1.

26. Corentin Gonthier, Lucie Longuépée, and Martine Bouvard, "Sensory Processing in Low-Functioning Adults with Autism Spectrum Disorder: Distinct Sensory Profiles and Their Relationships with Behavioral Dysfunction," *Journal of Autism and Developmental Disorders* 46, no. 9 (2016): 3,078–3,089, https://doi.org/10.1007/s10803-016-2850-1.

27. Kranowitz, *The Out-Of-Sync Child*.

28. Yasuda et al., "Sensory Cognitive Abnormalities of Pain in ASD."

29. Wanqing Zhang, Grace Baranek, and Brian Boyd, "Brief Report: Factors Associated with Emergency Department Visits for Epilepsy among Children with Autism Spectrum Disorder," *Journal of Autism and Developmental Disorders* 48, no. 5 (2017): 1,854–1,860, https://doi.org/10.1007/s10803-017-3433-5; and Roberto F. Tuchman, "Treatment of Seizure Disorders and EEG Abnormalities in Children with Autism Spectrum Disorders," *Journal of Autism and Developmental Disorders* 30, no. 5 (2000): 485–489.

30. Hirokazu Oguni, "Epilepsy and Intellectual and Developmental Disabilities," *Journal of Policy and Practice in Intellectual Disabilities* 10, no. 2 (2013): 89–92, https://doi.org/10.1111/jppi.12035.

31. Zhang et al., "Brief Report: Factors Associated with Emergency Department Visits."

32. Lori McIlwain and Wendy Fournier, "Lethal Outcomes in Autism Spectrum Disorders: Wandering/Elopement," National Autism Association, January 20, 2012, retrieved April 21, 2018, http://nationalautismassociation.org/wp-content/uploads/2012/01/Lethal-Outcomes-In-Autism-Spectrum-Disorders_2012.pdf; Bridget Kiely et al., "Prevalence and Correlates of Elopement in a Nationally Representative Sample of Children with Developmental Disabilities in the United States," *PLoS ONE* 11, no. 2 (2016): 1–11, https://doi.org/10.1371/journal.pone.0148337; and Catherine Rice et al., "Reported Wandering Behavior among Children with Autism Spectrum Disorder and/or Intellectual Disability," *Journal of Pediatrics* 174 (2016): 232–239, https://doi.org/10.1016/j.jpeds.2016.03.047.

33. Paul Law and Connie Anderson, "IAN Research Report: Elopement and Wandering," April 20, 2011, retrieved May 18, 2018, https://iancommunity.org/cs/ian_research_reports/ian_research_report_elopement.

34. Law and Anderson, "IAN Research Report."

35. McIlwain and Fournier, "Lethal Outcomes in Autism Spectrum Disorders."

36. Lori McIlwain, "Autism and Wandering: A Guide for First Responders," April 20, 2015, retrieved July 11, 2017, http://nationalautismassociation.org/autism-wandering-a-guide-for-first-responders/.

3

Intellectual Disabilities

Louise is a 43-year-old, morbidly obese woman with a profound intellectual disability and a diagnosis of Down syndrome. Her elderly parents called 911 because Louise was typically ambulatory but had refused to stand or walk for the last 12 hours. They believed, due to a history of abdominal issues, that she was experiencing abdominal pain, but they were unable to explain precisely why they thought she was in pain. Louise had been seen at the emergency department three days prior with a similar complaint but had been discharged with no diagnosis or resolution of her symptoms.

You enter the residence and locate your patient, sitting on the floor watching you, frowning, grunting (but not speaking), and clutching a well-worn stuffed dog. As you reach down to lift Louise to the stretcher, she screams, frantically scoots out of your reach, goes limp, and then swats and kicks at your crew as they attempt to help her. You ask the family if there is anything that calms her, and they say that she loves the Christmas song, "Rudolph, the Red-Nosed Reindeer." Even though it is 85°F outside on this summer day, you start singing and encourage your crew to do the same. Soon Louise is calmer and is able to be helped to the stretcher. She is uneventfully transported to the hospital with her sister next to her in the ambulance. In the emergency department, examination and imaging reveal that Louise had been swallowing the plastic lids off soda bottles. Emergency surgery recovers more than 50 bottle lids in her stomach.

While the term *intellectual disability (ID)* might be unfamiliar, it is simply an updated term for what used to be called *mental retardation*. In 2010, Rosa's Law (Public Law 111-256) was signed by former President Barack Obama. This law called for replacing the term *mental retardation* with *intellectual*

47

disability in federal health, education, and labor policies. While intellectual disability is the only appropriate term for professionals to use when describing individuals with developmentally impaired cognitive functioning, you may still hear family members, especially older family members, using the outdated term.

The American Association of Intellectual and Developmental Disabilities (AAIDD) defines an intellectual disability as "a disability characterized by significant limitations in both intellectual functioning and in adaptive behavior, which covers many everyday social and practical skills. This disability originates before the age of 18."[1]

The American Psychiatric Association states that "Intellectual Disability (Intellectual/Developmental Disorder) is a disorder with onset during the developmental period that includes both intellectual and adaptive functioning deficits in conceptual, social, and practical domains."[2] The APA definition notes that deficits in intellectual or cognitive functioning include problems with language, memory, reasoning, problem-solving, planning, abstract thinking, judgment, academic learning, and learning from experience. Deficits in adaptive functioning include not meeting developmental, social, and cultural standards for independence and social responsibility. The impact of these deficits limit functioning in the activities of daily life, including communication, interaction in society, and independent living, at home, school, work, and recreational activities.[3]

Although the definitions from the AAIDD and APA do not provide quantitative mandates or test score requirements for what constitutes deficits in intellectual and adaptive functioning, the AAIDD notes that both the intellectual and adaptive limitations criteria must be met through standardized testing.[4] First the individual must have a cognitive ability or intelligence quotient (IQ) as measured by a traditional IQ test at or below 70 to 75 points, or at least two standard deviations below the mean of 100. (The average IQ range is between 90 and 109 points.) In addition to the IQ criterion, individuals must also have limitations/difficulties with adaptive behaviors and functioning, with standardized adaptive functioning test scores at least two standard deviations below the mean, or less than or equal to 70 points. It is estimated that those who have an intellectual disability represent less than 2% of the US population.[5]

Identification of Intellectual Disability

Cognitive ability

Cognition is defined as "a broad range of largely invisible activities carried out by the human brain."[6] These activities include "perceiving, thinking, knowing, reasoning, remembering, analyzing, planning, paying attention, generating and synthesizing ideas, creating, judging, being aware, [and] having insight."[7] As an individual's cognitive ability of an individual encompasses a variety of skills, individuals with an intellectual disability can have challenges in multiple areas, not just verbal (spoken language) and nonverbal abilities. Cognitive functioning is measured in several domains, including verbal reasoning, general knowledge and comprehension, vocabulary, visual-spatial reasoning, perception, processing speed, and memory. Psychomotor abilities are also measured, including fine and gross muscle speed, strength, and movement, as well as coordination, manipulation, and dexterity.[8]

Adaptive behaviors

Adaptive behaviors are conceptual, social, and practical skills needed by all individuals to function in everyday life. These skill competencies and expectations vary by age level. Young children are not expected to have the same level of adaptive behaviors as their elders, regardless of cognitive ability. As children mature into adults, they are expected to be able to perform more and increasingly complex self-care behaviors independently.

These skills include the following:

- *Conceptual/language skills.* Literacy, money, time, self-direction, reasoning, learning from experience, etc.
- *Social/interpersonal interaction skills.* The ability to make and sustain friendships, empathy, social judgment, self-esteem, responsibility, rule following, self-protection (avoiding being victimized), etc.
- *Practical skills.* Activities of daily living (dressing, feeding, hygiene, toileting, mobility), money management, safety, occupational/vocational tasks, transportation, schedules, etc.[9]

Causes of Intellectual Disability

Intellectual disabilities have various prenatal and postnatal causes. Prenatal causes of ID include those with a chromosomal basis, such as Down syndrome, Prader-Willi syndrome, and fragile X syndrome (covered in more detail later in the chapter); maternal illnesses like rubella, toxoplasmosis, and group B strep; and inherited metabolic disorders, such as Tay-Sachs disease and phenylketonuria (PKU). Nongenetic prenatal and postnatal causes of ID include fetal alcohol spectrum disorders, birth trauma, significant prematurity, low birth weight, lead poisoning, near drowning, and traumatic brain injuries from accidents or shaken baby syndrome. An intellectual disability must manifest in the developmental period (before the age of 18 years). Note that many causes of ID are associated with medical and/or psychiatric comorbidities (discussed in more detail below).

While some types of intellectual disabilities cannot be avoided, like those caused by genetic disorders, others can be prevented. Fetal alcohol syndrome (discussed below) can be entirely prevented through maternal abstinence of alcohol during pregnancy. Passing group B strep from mother to newborn can be halted by maternal testing at 35 to 37 weeks gestation, which is followed by maternal antibiotics during labor if positive.[10] Other risk factors, such as poverty, maternal and infant/child malnutrition, environmental toxins, lack of access to prenatal care and preventative medicine, and child abuse, can be mediated. Exposure to these risk factors, however, does not predict whether an individual will or will not develop an intellectual disability.[11]

Classification of Intellectual Disability

The average IQ range is 90–109, with scores above 130 being in the upper extreme range and under 70 in the lower extreme range. In the past, severity levels of intellectual disability were determined by an individual's IQ.

Levels of intellectual disability severity are now more appropriately classified based on the adaptive functioning of the individuals and how much support they need from others in the conceptual, social, and practical domains (table 3–1). The APA (in DSM-5) and AAIDD both suggest expectations for individuals with ID with regards to their adaptive functioning in order to determine the severity of their condition.[12] Each person with ID has unique strengths and weaknesses, so an individual may "split" categories depending on which attribute is being considered.

Table 3–1. Severity of intellectual disability

Severity	AAIDD[*] Based on amount and intensity of support provided by others	DSM-5[†] Based on daily living skills and independence
Mild	Intermittent support • Supports provided as needed • Increased need typically during periods of transition • Can vary in intensity	• May have age-appropriate skills in personal care and recreation skills • May need additional support for health and legal decisions • May have competitive employment opportunities • May be able to live independently with minimal support
Moderate	Limited support • Supports are consistent or provided regularly over time but are time-limited (e.g., short-term)	• Needs regular assistance with daily tasks, including self-care, but task independence is possible • Employment opportunities require consistent and frequent support from others • May benefit from supported housing (group home setting)
Severe	Extensive support • Supports are regular • May be provided in multiple environments • Supports are not time-limited (e.g., they are long-term)	• Has limited verbal communication • Requires support and supervision for all daily and self-care activities • May exhibit self-injurious behaviors • Cannot make responsible decisions
Profound	Pervasive support • Supports are constant and of high intensity • Supports are provided across multiple environments • May be of a life-sustaining nature	• Fully dependent on others for all care at all times • May have sensory and/or physical impairments as well • Minimal verbal communication/speech • May exhibit self-injurious behaviors

Sources:

[*] American Association on Mental Retardation, *Mental Retardation: Definition, Classification, and Systems of Supports*, 10th ed. (Washington, DC: AAMR, 2002), 152.

[†] American Psychiatric Association, *Diagnostic and Statistical Manual of Mental Disorders*, 5th ed., DSM–5 (Washington, DC: American Psychiatric Association, 2013): 34–36.

General Considerations When Treating Patients with an Intellectual Disability

Challenges with communication

Individuals with intellectual disabilities may have communication delays or impaired communication. Consequently, it can be difficult not only to understand what they might be communicating to you but also to determine if they understand what you are communicating to them. The degree of communication challenges will be directly related to the severity of the intellectual disability. Some individuals with a severe intellectual disability may be unable to communicate effectively.

The Developmental Disabilities Primary Care Program, located in Toronto, Canada, publishes "Tools for the Primary Care of People with Developmental Disabilities," which provides excellent guidelines for communicating with people who have intellectual disabilities and ensuring that you obtain informed consent before administering care (see table 3–2). While this publication is designed for healthcare providers in an office setting (physicians, physician assistants, nurse practitioners, etc.), their suggestions can be adapted for the prehospital setting.

Table 3–2. Suggestions for communicating more effectively with patients with intellectual and developmental disabilities

Communicating Effectively with People Who Have Intellectual and Developmental Disabilities

- People with intellectual/developmental disabilities are likely to have communication difficulties.
- It will generally take more time to communicate.
- An assessment of language skills helps you choose the level of language to use. Talking with someone who has a mild intellectual/developmental disability is very different than talking with a person who has a moderate or severe intellectual/developmental disability.
- Many people with intellectual/developmental disabilities have stronger receptive (understanding) communication skills than expressive skills. Assume that the person with intellectual/developmental disabilities can understand more than he or she can communicate.
- Conversely, the person's expressive speech may sometimes give an impression of better comprehension than is actually the case, so check the person's understanding.

Table 3–2. ...*continued*

- People with intellectual/developmental disabilities have a variable, and sometimes limited, ability to interpret their internal cues (e.g., need to urinate, anxiety). They may not be able to give you an accurate picture of their feelings and symptoms. Involving caregivers who know the person well may help you to better understand his or her subjective experiences. However, continue to focus your communication efforts on the person rather than his or her caregiver.
- If you are in a busy area with many distractions, consider moving to a quieter location to minimize environmental distraction.

Goal	Suggested Communication Tips
Establishing rapport	• Speak directly to the person with developmental disabilities, not to his or her caregiver(s). • Ask the person, "Do you want your support worker/family member to stay here for this visit?" • Explain at the outset the purpose and process of the meeting in simple terms. • Ask simple introductory questions (e.g., name, reason for visit). • Gain the person's attention and eye contact if possible by using his or her name or by touching the person's arm prior to speaking. • Determine how they communicate: "How do you say yes or no?" "Do you use a device?" "Can you show me how to use this book/machine?" • If the person uses a communication technique or device, involve a caregiver who is familiar with it. • Show warmth and a positive regard. • Encourage the use of "comforters" (e.g., a favorite item the person likes to carry or a preference for standing and pacing rather than sitting). • Show interest in a precious object the person is holding on to. • Some people prefer to avoid eye contact. This should be respected. • Use positive reinforcement and focus on the person's abilities rather than disabilities.

Table 3–2. ...*continued*

Choosing appropriate language	• Use plain language. Avoid jargon.
	• Use short, simple sentences.
	• Use concrete as opposed to abstract language, such as the following: "Show me," "Tell me," "Do this" (with gesture), "Now," "Come with me," and/or "I'm going to…"
	• Use specific instructions such as, "Put your coat on" instead of "Get ready."
	• Use "Are you upset?" "Are you sad?" or "Are you happy?" instead of "What are you feeling?"
	• The concept of time is abstract and may be difficult to comprehend. Use examples from daily and familiar routines (e.g., breakfast, lunch, dinner, bedtime).
Listening	• Let the person know when you have understood them.
	• Be sensitive to cues and tone of voice.
	• It may be difficult to read facial expressions or body language because of differences in muscle tone. You may need to check/validate your perceptions.
	• Tell the person when you do not understand him or her.
	• Be aware that the visit will likely take more time than usual and that several consultations may be required to complete a full assessment.
Explaining clearly	• Speak slowly. Do not shout.
	• Pause frequently, so as not to overload the person with words.
	• Give the person with intellectual/developmental disabilities enough time to understand what you have said and to respond.
	• Rephrase and repeat questions if necessary, or write them out.
	• Check understanding. Ask the person, "Can you explain what I just said?" "Can you explain what I am going to do and why?"
	• If you are unsure whether the person has understood, ask, "Can you repeat what I said in your own words?"

Table 3–2. *...continued*

Commu- nicating without words	• People with poor language understanding rely on routines and cues from their environment to understand or anticipate what will happen. • Use pictures or simple diagrams and gestures (e.g., basic sign language). • Some people with intellectual/developmental disabilities may express themselves only in writing. • Allow them to handle and explore equipment. • Act out actions or procedures. • Use picture language when explaining; find signs in their communication book, saying, "It looks like..." (point to objects familiar to the person with intellectual/developmental disabilities). • Point to a body part or mime a procedure (e.g., checking ears).

Source: Adapted from the Developmental Disabilities Primary Care Program (DDPCP), *Tools for the Primary Care of People with Developmental Disabilities and Primary Care of Adults with Developmental Disabilities: Canadian Consensus Guidelines* (Toronto: Surrey Place Centre, 2011), http://www.surreyplace.ca/. All tools © 2011 Surrey Place Centre.

Obtaining informed consent/assent for assessment and treatment

Due to the challenges with communication and the potential for misunderstanding and confusion on the part of both the patient and the provider, it is difficult to know if the individual with ID has the capacity to make informed decisions about their care and is able to consent to care. While it is important to follow local laws, EMS protocols, and department policy about when to insist on transport or when to accept a refusal of care, the suggestions from the Developmental Disabilities Primary Care Program in table 3–3 can help you determine if the individual can make medical decisions for themselves. Note that these suggestions for determining capacity and informed consent can apply to other disabilities, including autism spectrum disorders, mental illness, and some physical disabilities.

Table 3–3. Determining capacity and obtaining consent

Determining Capacity*

Capacity refers to the mental ability to make a particular decision at a particular time. It is question- and decision-specific and should be documented relative to each decision. Assess capacity to consent for each treatment or plan of treatment. Even when a power of attorney (POA) for medical care exists, capacity for consent to the particular treatment at this time should be assessed.

- Capacity is not static but can change over time or require distinct abilities depending on the nature and complexity of the specific treatment decision. Specific capabilities may be lost or gained at different times during the life of a patient with intellectual/developmental disabilities. Situations may arise where consent to a treatment has been given or refused on a patient's behalf. However, if that patient then becomes capable of consenting to the treatment in the opinion of the health care practitioner, the patient's own decision would take precedence over that of the authorized decision maker.

- Assessed capacity can vary according to the supports provided. Involve the patient whenever possible by adapting the level and means of communicating to him or her. Patients require functionally appropriate means of communication and support to realize their capacity for informed consent to, or refusal of, treatment. Offer information in a form you believe the patient will understand (e.g., pictures, symbols, gestures, vignettes). (See also table 3–2)

- Involve others who know the patient best, such as family members or paid caregivers, to obtain information or to facilitate the patient's understanding and communication.

- If the patient is incapable of giving consent, or if there is uncertainty in this regard, follow appropriate legal procedures and ethical guidelines for assessing capacity. If incapable, delegate authority for decision making, which should be based on the patient's best interests in the circumstances. Generally only patients with mild to moderate intellectual/developmental disabilities will be capable of consenting, whereas those with severe to profound intellectual/developmental disabilities will not have that capability but may be able to assent to a proposed treatment. Whenever possible, even when consent is obtained from an authorized decision maker, assent from the patient should be sought and documented.

Table 3–3. ...*continued*

Obtaining and Documenting Consent*

- Consent must be given voluntarily.
  - Allow sufficient time for the patient to understand, consider the information, and ask questions.
  - If the patient requests additional information, provide a timely response.
- Consent must be related to a proposed investigation or treatment and be informed by adequate disclosure.
  - The EMS provider obtaining consent should be knowledgeable and well-informed about the condition and proposed intervention.
- Consent must not be obtained through fraud, coercion, or misrepresentation.
  - The patient should not be under any duress or pain.
  - It is important to be familiar with how the individual with intellectual/developmental disabilities usually exhibits pain (e.g., normal or unique pain responses), which may unduly affect decisions.

*Note: These are general suggestions only. Always refer to local laws and policies.

Source: Adapted from the Developmental Disabilities Primary Care Program (DDPCP), *Tools for the Primary Care of People with Developmental Disabilities and Primary Care of Adults with Developmental Disabilities: Canadian Consensus Guidelines* (Toronto: Surrey Place Centre, 2011), http://www.surreyplace.ca/. All tools © 2011 Surrey Place Centre.

Even if your patient is legally unable to consent because someone else has the legal authority to make decisions on his or her behalf, it is important to attempt to obtain an individual's assent to touch them or transport them to the hospital. *Assent* is simply agreeing to something. While a family member or caregiver may have legal decision-making authority for a person with an intellectual/developmental disability, it is still kind and appropriate to ask the person, "Is it okay if I touch you?" before conducting your assessment or performing any interventions.

Some additional questions to help determine an individual's capacity to make decisions on their own behalf include the following:[13]

- *Does the patient understand the information?* You can ask them to repeat back what you said in their own words.
- *Can the patient retain the information?* If they have memory deficits, you can provide written material or encourage them to write down the information you are providing.

- *Can they use the information you have provided to make decisions?* Some people become overwhelmed and anxious when presented with a lot of information at once. Do they comprehend the implications of their choices?
- *Are they able to communicate their decisions to you?* Are they able to speak or write their decision in a way that you are clear about their wishes?

It is also important to remember that capacity and consent ideally should be obtained with each new procedure or dissemination of new information, and that capacity to consent can change over time and/or may be impacted or influenced by the presenting issues.[14] Although the care and treatment of the individual is a priority and the urgency of their health needs might ultimately override their preferences, being respectful and working toward establishing a rapport and gaining their assent can, in the long run, save time and facilitate your assessment and treatment.

If an authorized caregiver gives consent for assessment and treatment, be sure to explain to the caregiver what you intend to do and why you want to do it, but also do not forget to explain in developmentally appropriate terms to the patient as well, even if you are unsure as to how much they understand.

Suggested questions from the Developmental Disabilities Primary Care Program that you can consider asking as additional support for determining capacity and obtaining informed consent are provided in table 3–4. Answering yes or no to these questions may not necessarily indicate an individual's ability to consent but can help as you talk with your patient.

As always, consult local authorities or legal guidance specific to your area or jurisdiction.

Table 3–4. Suggested questions for obtaining informed, voluntary consent

Suggested Questions for Obtaining Informed, Voluntary Consent
Does the patient understand that you are offering an intervention for a health problem?
– What problems are you having right now?
– What problem is bothering you most?
– Do you know why you are in the hospital/clinic?

Table 3–4. ...*continued*

Does the patient understand the nature of the proposed investigation or treatment and the expected benefits, burdens, and risks?

- What could be done to help you with your (specify health problem)?
- Do you think you are able to have this treatment?
- Do you know what might happen to you if you have this treatment?
- Do you know if this treatment can cause problems? Can it help you live longer?

Does the patient understand possible alternative treatment options and their expected benefits, burdens, and risks?

- Do you know different ways that might make you better?

Does the patient understand the likely effects of not having the proposed investigation or treatment?

- Do you know what could happen to you if you don't have this (specify the procedure or treatment) done?
- Could you get sicker or die if you don't have this (specify the treatment or procedure)?
- Do you know what could happen if you have this (specify the treatment or procedure)?

Is the patient free from any duress (e.g., illness, family pressure), pain, or distress that might impair his or her capacity regarding the particular decision? (Note that a relatively minor illness can cause significant anxiety.)

- Can you help me understand why you've decided to accept/refuse this treatment?
- Is anyone telling you that you should or should not get this treatment?

Is the patient free from a mental health condition (e.g., mood disturbance or psychiatric illness) that may influence his or her capacity to give consent? (Note that having a mental health condition is not in itself an indicator of permanent incapacity. This factor may change once the mental health condition is treated.)

- Are you hopeful about the future?
- Do you think you deserve to be treated?
- Do you think anyone is trying to hurt and/or harm you?
- Do you trust the people who are here to help you?

Table 3–4. ...*continued*

- If the answer is yes to *all* of the above, and the patient can remember the information long enough to make a decision (verify by asking the patient to explain the information to you), *then consider that capability exists to consent to or refuse the proposed treatment.*

- If the answer is no to *any* of the above, then repeat the questions. You may need to repeat this process several times to ensure that the patient understands. If the patient still does not understand, *he or she is incapable, and an authorized decision maker should provide consent.*

- If you are unsure about any of the above or if decision-making capacity is present, consult family members, caregivers, or law enforcement present for guidance, or contact medical control per jurisdictional policies for guidance and/or orders.

Source: Adapted from the Developmental Disabilities Primary Care Program (DDPCP), *Tools for the Primary Care of People with Developmental Disabilities and Primary Care of Adults with Developmental Disabilities: Canadian Consensus Guidelines* (Toronto: Surrey Place Centre, 2011), http://www.surreyplace.ca/. All tools © 2011 Surrey Place Centre.

Pain

As stated above, some causes of intellectual disability are associated with certain medical/psychiatric comorbidities (discussed in more detail below) that can place people with ID at a higher risk for experiencing pain than the general population. Pain is subjective and cannot be accurately measured by physiological markers or diagnostic tests. Ideally it is self-reported, but even a neurotypical person can have trouble describing and quantifying pain. Given the challenges inherent with impaired cognitive ability and language, as well as trouble with conceptualizing pain, patients with ID are at risk for having their pain misidentified and undertreated by their caregivers and health-care providers.[15]

Providing adequate pain management to patients with ID can be difficult as it may be hard to recognize their pain and its severity. Findlay et al. describe pain detection by others as an "art" as well as "complex and...ambiguous."[16]

Use caregivers as a resource in pain identification and assessing severity, as they know the patient best. Caregivers often report that while they tend to have the best knowledge of the patient, their concerns often go unheard.[17] Detecting and treating pain is important, not just because it is ethical and kind to mitigate someone's pain whenever possible, but also because pain, both chronic and acute, can contribute to behavioral issues that can be reduced when pain is decreased.[18]

Findlay et al. noted the following behaviors observed by caregivers as possible signs of pain.[19] They advised that overmedicating for perceived or real pain is dangerous and advised the use of caution (as well as other indicators) when interpreting these signs as indications of pain:

- *Vocalization.* Excessive talking, decreased talking, shouting, swearing.
- *Facial expressions.* Grimacing, squinting.
- *Behavior/movement.* Excessive sleeping, not sleeping, frequent waking, pacing, rocking, limping.
- *Aggression.* Towards others or self-injurious behaviors.
- *Emotions.* Crying, agitation, fear.
- *Physiological.* Fever, redness, sweating, swelling.

The use of other physiological signs may also be helpful when attempting to assess pain. An increase in blood pressure, respiratory rate, or heart rate over baseline can indicate pain but may also be indicative of other physiological processes, like having a bowel movement. Because pain is subjective, remember that your pain assessment will also be subjective.[20]

The Nonverbal Pain Scale (NVPS), developed by the University of Rochester, can be a useful tool when assessing patients who are nonverbal or who have limited communication abilities. This scale (see table 3–5) can help providers quantify pain through a five-item, 10-point scale, as well as help evaluate if a patient's pain is improving or worsening over time.

Booker and Haedtke provide suggestions for nurses who are assessing pain in hospitalized adults who may be unable to communicate due to ventilation, sedation, dementia, aphasia, or cognitive impairments.[21] While these suggestions have been designed for patients in the hospital, they can be adapted for providers in the prehospital setting.

Their first recommendation is to encourage self-report of pain by patients if at all possible. Patients who are nonverbal or have difficulty speaking might be able to write or draw a picture to indicate the location and/or severity of their pain.

Table 3–5. Adult Nonverbal Pain Scale

Adult Nonverbal Pain Scale			
Categories	**0**	**1**	**2**
Face	No particular expression or smile	Occasional grimace, tearing, frowning, wrinkled forehead	Frequent grimace, tearing, frowning, wrinkled forehead
Activity/ Movement	Lying quietly, normal position	Seeking attention through movement or slow, cautious movement	Restless, excessive activity, and/or withdrawal reflexes
Guarding	Lying quietly, no positioning of hands over areas of body	Splinting areas of the body, tense	Rigid, stiff
Physiology/ Vital Signs	Stable vital signs	Change in any of the following: * SBP > 20 mm Hg * HR > 20/min.	Change in any of the following: * SBP > 30 mm Hg * HR > 25/min.
Respiratory	Baseline RR/SpO$_2$ Compliant with ventilator	RR > 10 above baseline, or 5% ↓SpO$_2$ Mild asynchrony with ventilator	RR > 20 above baseline, or 10% ↓SpO$_2$ Severe asynchrony with ventilator

Abbreviations: HR, heart rate; RR, respiratory rate; SBP, systolic blood pressure; SpO$_2$, pulse oximetry.

Instructions: Each of the five categories is scored from 0 to 2, which results in a total score between 0 and 10. Document total score by adding numbers from each of the five categories. Scores of 0 to 2 indicate no pain; 3 to 6, moderate pain; and 7 to 10, severe pain.

Document assessment every four hours on nursing flowsheet and complete assessment before and after intervention to maximize patient comfort. Sepsis, hypovolemia, hypoxia need to be excluded before interventions.

Source: © 2003 University of Rochester. Used with permission.

The second step is to consider if there is a source of pain. Do they have a medical history or diagnosis that would cause pain, such as arthritis or a broken bone? Have they had a recent medical procedure that could cause pain, either as part of the procedure (stitches or recent surgery) or due to complications (such as a urinary tract infection following catheterization)? Are their clothes rubbing or pinching? If they have limited mobility and spend the majority of their time in bed or in a wheelchair, do they have a pressure ulcer?

The third step in Booker and Haedtke's recommendations is to look for behavioral and physiological indicators of pain.[22] As suggested above, these can include changes in facial expressions, agitation, anxiety, crying, and changes in typical behavior, as well as changes in vital signs. They caution, however, against using vital signs alone as a pain determinant as patients may already be on medications such as antihypertensives or antidysrhythmics, which can influence the impact of pain on vital signs.[23] People with chronic pain or acute and chronic pain may not have changes in vital signs.[24] Regular caregivers such as family members, residence staff, and home health nurses can provide valuable information with regards to changes in behavior, and what constitutes baseline vital signs and behaviors.

Once it is believed that the patient is experiencing pain, a pain management trial can be implemented, starting with nonopioid pain control, if available, and moving to low dose opioids. Booker and Haedtke caution against using placebo attempts (saline flushes) or underdosing (unless advised to do so by medical control) as this will not control pain effectively.[25] While the final step in their pain assessment pathway is not practical for prehospital providers, their last recommendation is for the patient's healthcare team to develop a long-term pain treatment plan.

Findlay, Williams, and Scior conducted a small-scale investigation of how 15 people with intellectual disabilities experienced pain and how their pain was addressed by others.[26] This study revealed that some people with ID have a difficult time finding words to describe their pain effectively or may have pain that is not sufficiently communicated through behaviors other than verbal language. This can lead to pain being overrated or underrated by the patients, making pain management challenging. While the problems associated with underrating pain are obvious—the patient might not get effective pain management—there are risks with overrating pain as well. Providers across the spectrum (home, prehospital, and hospital) may believe that the pain is exaggerated and might not take the patient seriously. People with ID also reported that they sometimes hid that they were in pain in an effort to avoid potentially unpleasant consequences (trips to the doctor or ED, swallowing pills, needles from IVs/injections). The authors of this study provided the following recommendations when assessing the pain levels of someone with an intellectual disability:

- Be cautious with the questions that are asked and how they are asked (leading, yes/no, etc.).

- Recognize that pain can lead to challenging behaviors.

- Use pictures when possible but recognize that the commonly used face rating scale may not be reliable due to ambiguity in the meaning of the different faces, especially the smiling face.

- Understand that just because a person can communicate verbally does not mean that they can effectively communicate about their pain severity.

Assessing pain can be challenging even when working with patients without intellectual disabilities and communication challenges. Being able to assess and relieve someone's pain, however, is not only ethical and kind, it can make your job easier and safer.

Agitation and aggressive behavior

Individuals with an intellectual disability are at increased risk for displaying agitated and aggressive behavior, which can pose a significant risk for EMS responders. This can be compounded by the individual's challenges with communication and cognitive understanding of a situation. In a study of almost 300 adults with ID, Crocker et al. found that almost 87% had demonstrated aggressive behavior.[27] Verbal aggression toward others was the most commonly displayed behavior (77%), followed by property aggression (62.5%), physical aggression (55%), and sexual aggression (20%). Incidences of these behaviors were fairly evenly divided between men and women. Other items of note include the following:

- Individuals with a moderate intellectual disability were at almost twice the risk of displaying physical aggression as those with a mild intellectual disability.

- Additional diagnoses of mental health disorders increased the incidence of verbal and property aggression.

Many individuals with an intellectual disability who display aggressive behaviors will need to be transported to the emergency department for evaluation and treatment, and you may be called (along with law enforcement) to assess and transport. Be especially cognizant and aware that a patient who is not initially aggressive, or one that you might not typically consider likely to be aggressive, can become so without much warning.

Pica

Pica is the eating of nonfood items (paper, chalk, dirt, cigarette butts, hair, etc.) and/or nonnutritive items (flour, lard, ice, spoiled/discarded food, dog food, etc.) that persists for more than one month and is not part of a culturally accepted practice.[28] Children under the age of two years typically will not receive a pica diagnosis because it is developmentally appropriate for infants and toddlers, even those without intellectual disabilities, to put nonfood items in their mouths and potentially swallow them.

Pica can occur as a stand-alone diagnosis in the absence of another disorder or as comorbid with another disorder, such as an intellectual disability or an autism spectrum disorder. It is relatively common in people with an intellectual disability and in one study was observed in 22% of institutionalized adults with an intellectual disability.[29]

The health risks of pica are serious and therefore are of particular interest to EMS providers who may encounter a patient having a significant medical complication as a result. *Coprophagia*, or eating of feces, can result in parasitic or bacterial infections, such as worms or *E. coli*. An intestinal blockage can occur from a *bezoar*, which is a mass of indigestible material, sometimes caused by eating hair, fabric, or carpet.[30] Other possible complications from eating nonfood or nonnutritional material include ulcers, gastrointestinal bleeding, gastrointestinal perforation, and lead toxicity (from eating metal, paint, or soil).[31]

EMS providers will want to consider any of these possible complications when assessing a patient with an intellectual disability, especially if the chief complaint involves abdominal pain, nausea, or vomiting, or you have reason to believe the patient engages in pica. It is also important that you ensure that your patient does not have the opportunity to eat anything from the ambulance such as gauze, bandages, or electrodes.

Some Types of Intellectual Disability with Special Considerations for EMS

Down syndrome

Down syndrome is one of the oldest recognized and best-known causes of intellectual disabilities, with evidence of the condition seen in works of art dating from more than 3,000 years ago (figs. 3–1 and 3–2).[32] The condition was formally described by John Langdon Down in 1866 but was not given his name until the 1970s.

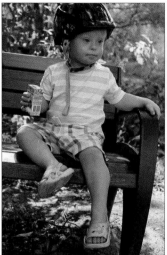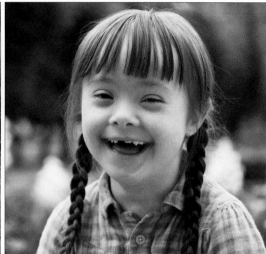

Figs. 3–1 and 3–2. Down syndrome is the oldest and best-known cause of intellectual disability.
Courtesy: Pixabay.com.

Although there are several underlying genetic mutations that cause Down syndrome, the most common cause, trisomy 21, occurs when the 21st chromosome is a trio, or "trisomy," instead of the typical pair of chromosomes. Down syndrome is more common in babies born to mothers over 40, increasing from fewer than 1 in 1,000 births in mothers in their 20s to 1 in 97 in mothers over 40.[33] The overall prevalence is 8 per 10,000 births in the United States, or just over 250,000 people.[34]

In addition to varying degrees of severity of intellectual disability (typically moderate to severe), Down syndrome has several physical characteristics that are common to individuals with the condition. People with Down syndrome have specific facial characteristics including a small, flattened nose, eyes that turn upward, and a tongue that appears large due to a smaller mouth/oral cavity. Additional physical characteristics include low muscle tone, hands/fingers that are smaller, and a tendency to be shorter in stature. They are at higher risk for being overweight or obese, with a subsequent increased risk for type II diabetes.[35]

In addition to diabetes, people with Down syndrome have higher rates of several other potentially serious health problems that should be considered during an EMS assessment including the following:

- Heart defects[36]
- Gastrointestinal problems, including reflux and celiac disease[37]
- Feeding and swallowing problems, due to oral structural and motor difficulties[38]
- Leukemia[39]
- Vision problems, including near-sightedness and far-sightedness, *strabismus* (crossed eyes), and cataracts[40]
- Hearing loss, including increased risk of otitis media (middle ear infections)[41]
- Hypothyroidism[42]
- Seizures[43]
- Early onset dementia[44]
- Sleep disorders, including sleep apnea and behavioral sleep disturbances[45]
- Musculoskeletal problems, including degenerative changes in the cervical spine, structural bone differences, and laxity and instability of ligaments[46]

Prader-Willi syndrome

Prader-Willi syndrome is a genetic condition occurring in 1 in 15,000 births and is caused by missing genes on the 15th chromosome.[47] Most people with Prader-Willi syndrome have a mild intellectual disability and academic skills below what is expected for their cognitive ability. Characteristic physical features in people with Prader-Willi syndrome include *hypotonia* (low muscle tone), almond-shaped eyes, a narrow forehead, smaller than average hands or feet, underdeveloped genitals, and short stature. Behavior problems are common with Prader-Willi syndrome, including temper tantrums, stubborn and resistant behavior, obsessions and compulsions, and skin-picking.[48]

The most unusual and central characteristic, however, is an insatiable appetite and chronic overeating that leads to obesity. The majority (87% in one report) of people with Prader-Willi syndrome are obese or morbidly obese,[49] with the health concerns associated with obesity, such as diabetes, hypertension, and sleep apnea. In the first few years of life, children with Prader-Willi syndrome often experience poor muscle tone, feeding problems, and failure to thrive.[50] Beginning around the ages of two to six years, children with Prader-Willi syndrome begin to demonstrate compulsive overeating, which is caused by deficits in the hypothalamus region of the brain that controls appetite and *satiety*, or the feeling of being full after eating. As they get older, subsequent behaviors associated with the acquisition of food emerge, including rummaging through the garbage, stealing food and stealing money to buy food, and leaving home unsupervised to look for food.[51] While this condition is separate from pica (discussed above), the same recommendations apply. When assessing a patient for abdominal pain or suspected toxic ingestion, consider that they may have eaten something they should not have. Be sure to secure items in the ambulance that can be consumed.

Fragile X syndrome

Fragile X syndrome, first clinically identified in 1943,[52] is a common genetic cause of intellectual disability, occurring in 1 in 4,000 males and 1 in 6,000 females.[53] The disorder is not only more prevalent in males, the clinical presentation tends to be more severe in males as well. Fragile X is a heritable disorder, with non-clinically affected mothers (carriers) passing the disorder onto their children.[54] Common physical characteristics include the following:[55]

- Intellectual disability
- Elongated face
- High, arched palate
- Large, protruding ears
- Enlarged testicles (*macroorchidism*)
- Flexible joints

Females with fragile X typically do not exhibit the common physical characteristics and may have intellectual abilities ranging from mild disability to average intelligence. They also may experience difficulties with math, motor skills, and speech/language, along with social problems and anxiety.[56]

Behavior

Behavior problems associated with both males and females with fragile X are common and can be significant. These behaviors include hyperactivity, impulsivity, tantrums, explosive behavior, self-injury, and aggression.[57] Fragile X is also one of the few known genetic causes of autism spectrum disorders, seen in as many as 30% to 50% of individuals with ASD,[58] and is associated with the common behavior characteristics of ASD outlined in chapter 2.

Wheeler et al. reported specifically on aggressive behavior associated with people who have fragile X syndrome.[59] They interviewed the caregivers of 774 individuals with fragile X and found that more than 90% of males and 80% of females had exhibited mild to moderate aggressive behaviors in the previous 12 months. The behaviors demonstrated were tantrums, defiance, arguing, and physical aggression (hitting, kicking, pushing), sometimes resulting in injury to caregivers (in 30% of study participants) and to friends and peers (22% of study participants), which is something to be remembered by EMS providers. The authors speculated that these aggressive behaviors were often precipitated by hypersensitivity to sensory stimuli (as seen in people with ASD and sensory processing disorder (SPD), discussed in detail in chapter 2).

As with patients with a primary diagnosis of ASD without fragile X, providers who are treating individuals with fragile X and associated ASD/SPD will want to remember that people with an unusual response to sensory stimuli may react unpredictably or aggressively.

Seizures

Seizures are also associated with fragile X syndrome. The prevalence of seizures/epilepsy in children worldwide is estimated at about 3 to 6 out of 1,000,[60] but in people with fragile X, it is considerably higher, with around 12% experiencing seizures.[61]

While severe seizures are not common in fragile X syndrome, there is one report in the literature reviewing instances in which five children (ages 5 to 14 years) experienced *status epilepticus* with their first seizure.[62] Status epilepticus has been traditionally defined as more than 30 minutes of seizure activity without stopping or two or more seizures in a 30-minute period without regaining consciousness. *Refractory status epilepticus* is a seizure that does not stop after pharmacological treatment.[63] Status epilepticus is potentially life-threatening due to respiratory depression and subsequent hypoxia. Singh et al. report a 20% mortality rate associated with status epilepticus, with the mortality rate of refractory status epilepticus significantly higher at 35%.[64] Benzodiazepines such as lorazepam, diazepam, or midazolam are the recommended first line of treatment and can be administered in the prehospital setting by family members or advanced life support (ALS) first responders.

Fetal alcohol spectrum disorders

Unlike Down syndrome, fragile X syndrome, and Prader-Willi syndrome, which are unpreventable genetic disorders that occur at the time of conception, fetal alcohol spectrum disorder is an environmental cause of intellectual disability that is entirely preventable. Maternal consumption of alcohol during pregnancy (even as little as one drink per week)[65] affects the developing fetus directly as a *teratogen*, a substance that can cause birth defects, and/or through the impact of alcohol consumption on the mother's health and lifestyle (e.g., poor nutrition, liver disease).

Fetal alcohol spectrum disorder is an umbrella term that includes the various severities of the disorder ranging from the most severe, fetal alcohol syndrome, to the least, neurodevelopmental disorder associated with alcohol exposure.[66]

Like other types of intellectual disabilities, fetal alcohol spectrum disorder has several distinctive physical, cognitive, and academic characteristics:[67]

- Flattened *philtrum* (the groove between the nose and the upper lip)
- Thin upper lip
- Small eyes
- Slow growth (height, weight, and head size)
- Average IQ less than 70
- Comorbid ADHD
- Social impairments
- Weakness in math skills
- Impaired memory
- Seizure disorder

- Poor theory of mind (See chapter 2 on autism spectrum disorders for a more in-depth discussion.)
- Executive functioning deficits
- Delayed language and poor language processing and comprehension
- Poor motor control and coordination
- Increased risk for behavior problems, including aggression and conduct disorder
- Increased risk for psychiatric disorders, including depression and panic disorder
- Reduced life expectancy (around 34 years compared to 79 to 83 years for the general population, depending on gender)

Conclusion

While it is impossible to predict how any individual will behave during an emergency situation, remember that when assessing and treating an individual with ID you may have problems with and should be prepared to address the following:

- Communication, including delayed speech and language
- Overstimulation and subsequent agitation
- Confusion, fear, and/or misunderstanding
- Sorting out the chief complaint and/or getting a complete history

Implications for EMS

- **Encourage family or caregivers to stay with the patient.** While your department will have guidelines about who can or cannot ride in the patient compartment of the ambulance, it will be to your advantage not to separate a patient with an intellectual disability from their caregiver if they appear anxious or fearful. Not only can the caregiver help you with assessment and understanding of the patient, they will also be able to act immediately as the patient's advocate. Additionally, many adults with an intellectual disability have a parent or other family member who holds a medical power of attorney with decision-making authority. Just as you would want a minor child's parents with them during transport and ED admission to be able to make medical decisions, you will also want an authorized decision maker present with an individual with an intellectual disability.

- **Use simple words and speak slowly.** This does not mean talking down to them, talking to them like they are a child (unless they are a child), or talking to them with exaggerated slowness, but it does mean choosing your words carefully and not using unnecessary medical terms or complicated, multipart questions. Ask one question at a time and wait for an answer before asking the next question.

- **Be cautious when assessing for pain.** Individuals with an intellectual disability, especially profound ID, may have difficulty communicating that they are in pain and how severe their pain is.[68]

- **Do not raise your voice unless they are hard of hearing.** A loud voice will not help them understand any better.

- **Be sensitive to nonverbal cues indicating anxiety or concern.** Especially in patients who have communication delays, your patient may be unable to articulate increasing worry or fear.

- **Use visuals (e.g., drawings) or gestures.** When possible, show or demonstrate before doing anything, even if it takes a little more time. You will ultimately save time by gaining the trust of your patient.

- **Explain everything before doing it, even if they appear not to understand.** People with an intellectual disability often can understand more than they can express or demonstrate, so tell them what you are going to do. Not only will this help the patient understand what you are going to do, it will also help the caregivers or family members know what to expect.

Notes

1. "Definition of Intellectual Disability," American Association on Intellectual and Developmental Disabilities, https://aaidd.org/intellectual-disability/definition#.WWzFnIjytEY.

2. American Psychiatric Association, *Diagnostic and Statistical Manual of Mental Disorders*, 5th ed., DSM–5 (Washington, DC: American Psychiatric Association, 2013): 33.

3. APA, *Diagnostic and Statistical Manual of Mental Disorders*.

4. American Association on Intellectual and Developmental Disabilities, *Intellectual Disability: Definition, Classification, and Systems of Supports*, 11th ed. (Washington, DC: AAIDD, 2010).

5. AAIDD, *Intellectual Disability*; APA, *Diagnostic and Statistical Manual of Mental Disorders*.

6. Soo Borson, "Cognition, Aging, and Disabilities: Conceptual Issues," *Physical Medicine and Rehabilitation Clinics of North America* 21, no. 2 (2010): 375, https://doi.org/10.1016/j.pmr.2010.01.001.

7. Borson, "Cognition, Aging, and Disabilities," 375.

8. APA, *Diagnostic and Statistical Manual of Mental Disorders*.

9. APA, *Diagnostic and Statistical Manual of Mental Disorders*; and Clifford J. Drew and Michael L. Hardman, *Intellectual Disabilities across the Lifespan*, 9th ed. (Upper Saddle River, NJ: Pearson Merrill Prentice Hall, 2007).

10. US Department of Health and Human Services, Centers for Disease Control and Prevention, "Prevention of Perinatal Group B Streptococcal Disease," Morbidity and Mortality Weekly Report 59, no. RR-10 (November 19, 2010): 1–36, https://www.cdc.gov/mmwr/pdf/rr/rr5910.pdf.

11. AAIDD, *Intellectual Disability*.

12. APA, *Diagnostic and Statistical Manual of Mental Disorders*; and AAIDD, *Intellectual Disability*.

13. Shelley Cummings, "How to Tell Whether Patients Can Make Decisions about Their Care," *Emergency Nurse* 20, no. 5 (2012): 22–26, https://doi.org/10.7748/en2012.09.20.5.22.c9289.

14. Cummings, "How to Tell Whether Patients Can Make Decisions about Their Care."

15. A. Amor-Salamanca and J. M. Menchon, "Pain Underreporting Associated with Profound Intellectual Disability in Emergency Departments," *Journal of Intellectual Disability Research* 61, no. 4 (2017): 341–347, https://doi.org/10.1111/jir.12355.

16. Laura Findlay et al., "Caregiver Experiences of Supporting Adults with Intellectual Disabilities in Pain," *Journal of Applied Research in Intellectual Disabilities* 28, no. 2 (2015): 111, 117, https://doi.org/10.1111/jar.12109.

17. Findlay et al., "Caregiver Experiences of Supporting Adults with Intellectual Disabilities in Pain."

18. I. Weissman-Fogel et al., "Pain Experience of Adults with Intellectual Disabilities—Caregiver Reports," *Journal of Intellectual Disability Research* 59, no. 10 (2015): 914–924, https://doi.org/:10.1111/jir.12194.

19. Findlay et al., "Caregiver Experiences of Supporting Adults with Intellectual Disabilities in Pain."

20. Mary Beth F. Makic, "Pain Management in the Nonverbal Critically Ill Patient," *Journal of PeriAnesthesia Nursing* 28, no. 2 (2013): 98–101, https://doi.org/10.1016/j.jopan.2013.01.006.

21. Staja Q. Booker and Christine Haedtke, "Assessing Pain in Nonverbal Older Adults," *Nursing* 46, no. 5 (2016): 66–69, https://doi.org/10.1097/01.nurse.0000480619.08039.50.

22. Booker and Haedtke, "Assessing Pain in Nonverbal Older Adults."

23. Makic, "Pain Management in the Nonverbal Critically Ill Patient."

24. P. Block et al., "Relations among Pain Variables and Vital Signs in Patients Presenting to the Emergency Department for Acute Pain, Exacerbations of Chronic Pain, and Acute Pain with Concurrent Chronic Pain," *The Journal of Pain* 15, no. 4 (2014): S18, https://doi.org/10.1016/j.jpain.2014.01.077.

25. Booker and Haedtke, "Assessing Pain in Nonverbal Older Adults."

26. Laura Findlay, Amanda C. de C. Williams, and Katrina Scior, "Exploring Experiences and Understandings of Pain in Adults with Intellectual Disabilities," *Journal of Intellectual Disability Research* 58, no. 4 (2014): 358–367, https://doi.org/10.1111/jir.12020.

27. Anne G. Crocker et al., "Intellectual Disability and Co-occurring Mental Health and Physical Disorders in Aggressive Behavior," *Journal of Intellectual Disability Research* 58, no. 11 (2014): 1,032–1,044, https://doi.org/10.1111/jir.12080.

28. APA, *Diagnostic and Statistical Manual of Mental Disorders*.

29. Melody Ashworth, Lynn Martin, and John P. Hirdes, "Prevalence and Correlates of Pica among Adults with Intellectual Disability in Institutions," *Journal of Mental Health Research in Intellectual Disabilities* 1, no. 3 (2008): 176–190, https://doi.org/10.1080/19315860802029154.

30. Zainab Ali, "Pica in People with Intellectual Disability: A Literature Review of Aetiology, Epidemiology and Complications," *Journal of Intellectual and Developmental Disability* 26, no. 2 (2001): 205–215, https://doi.org/10.1080/13668250020054486.

31. I. Kamal, J. Thompson, and D. M. Paquette, "The Hazards of Vinyl Glove Ingestion in the Mentally Retarded Patient with Pica: New Implications for Surgical Management," *Canadian Journal of Surgery* 42, no. 3 (1999): 210–204; Ali, "Pica in People with Intellectual Disability."

32. P. T. Rogers, M. Coleman, and S. Buckley, *Medical Care in Down Syndrome: A Preventive Medicine Approach* (New York, NY: Marcel Dekker, 1992).

33. Clifford J. Drew and Michael L. Hardman, *Intellectual Disabilities across the Lifespan* (Upper Saddle River, NJ: Pearson Merrill Prentice Hall, 2007).

34. A. P. Presson et al., "Current Estimate of Down Syndrome Population Prevalence in the United States," *Journal of Pediatrics* 163, no. 4 (2013): 1,163–1,168, https://doi.org/10.1016/j.jpeds.2013.06.013.

35. Robyn A. Wallace, "Clinical Audit of Gastrointestinal Conditions Occurring among Adults with Down Syndrome Attending a Specialist Clinic," *Journal of Intellectual and Developmental Disability* 32, no. 1 (2007): 45–50, https://doi.org/10.1080/13668250601146761; and Julie Murray and Patricia Ryan-Krause, "Obesity in Children with Down Syndrome: Background and Recommendations for Management," *Pediatric Nursing* 36, no. 6 (2010): 314–319.

36. Claudine Torfs and Roberta Christianson, "Maternal Risk Factors and Major Associated Defects in Infants with Down Syndrome," *Epidemiology* 10, no. 3 (1999): 264–270, https://doi.org/10.1097/00001648-199905000-00013.

37. Wallace, "Clinical Audit of Gastrointestinal Conditions Occurring among Adults with Down Syndrome Attending a Specialist Clinic"; and Geoffrey Holmes, "Gastrointestinal Disorders in Down Syndrome," *Gastroenterology and Hepatology from Bed to Bench* 7, no. 1 (2014): 6–8.

38. Linda Cooper-Brown et al., "Feeding and Swallowing Dysfunction in Genetic Syndromes," *Developmental Disabilities Research Reviews* 14, no. 2 (2008): 147–157, https://doi.org/10.1002/ddrr.19.

39. Irene Roberts and Shai Izraeli, "Haematopoietic Development and Leukaemia in Down Syndrome," *British Journal of Haematology* 167, no. 5 (2014): 587–599, https://doi.org/10.1111/bjh.13096.

40. Nabin Paudel et al., "Visual Defects in Nepalese Children with Down Syndrome," *Clinical and Experimental Optometry* 93, no. 2 (2010): 83–90, https://doi.org/10.1111/j.1444-0938.2010.00458.x; and Tanisha Watt, Kenneth Robertson, and Robert J. Jacobs, "Refractive Error, Binocular Vision and Accommodation of Children with Down Syndrome, *Clinical and Experimental Optometry* 98, no. 1 (2015): 3–11, https://doi.org/10.1111/cxo.12232.

41. N. J. Roizen et al., "Hearing Loss in Children with Down Syndrome," *Journal of Pediatrics* 123, no. 1 (1993): 9–12; and E. J. Glasson, D. E. Dye, and A. H. Bittles, "The Triple Challenges Associated with Age-Related Comorbidities in Down Syndrome," *Journal of Intellectual Disability Research* 58, no. 4 (2014): 393–398, https://doi.org/10.1111/jir.12026.

42. Murray and Ryan-Krause, "Obesity in Children with Down Syndrome"; Glasson, Dye, and Bittles, "The Triple Challenges."

43. G. Diaconu et al., "Epileptic Seizures in Children with Down Syndrome," *Romanian Journal of Pediatrics* 62, no. 1 (2013): 96–99.

44. Glasson, Dye, and Bittles, "The Triple Challenges Associated with Age-Related Comorbidities in Down Syndrome"; and Jin Chu, Thomas Wisniewski, and Domenico Praticò, "GATA1-Mediated Transcriptional Regulation of the γ-Secretase Activating Protein Increases Aβ Formation in Down Syndrome," *Annals of Neurology* 79, no. 1 (2016): 138–143, https://doi.org/10.1002/ana.24540.

45. A. J. Esbensen, "Sleep Problems and Associated Comorbidities Among Adults with Down Syndrome," *Journal of Intellectual Disability Research* 60, no. 1 (2016): 68–79, https://doi/10.1111/jir.12236.

46. Lynn Nadel and Donna Rosenthal, *Down Syndrome: Living and Learning in the Community* (New York: Wiley-Liss, 1995).

47. "PWS Basic Facts," Prader-Willi Syndrome Association-USA, http://www.pwsausa.org/.

48. E. M. Dykens, J. F. Leckman, and S. B. Cassidy, "Obsessions and Compulsions in Prader-Willi Syndrome," *Journal of Child Psychology and Psychiatry* 37, no. 8 (1996): 995–1,002; and S. E. McCandless, "Health Supervision for Children with Prader-Willi Syndrome," *Pediatrics* 127, no. 1 (2011): 195–204, https://doi.org/10.1542/peds.2010-2820.

49. V. Laurier et al., "Medical, Psychological and Social Features in a Large Cohort of Adults with Prader-Willi Syndrome: Experience from a Dedicated Centre in France," *Journal of Intellectual Disability Research* 59, no. 5 (2014): 411–421, https://doi.org/10.1111/jir.12140.

50. Cooper-Brown et al., "Feeding and Swallowing Dysfunction in Genetic Syndromes."

51. McCandless, "Health Supervision for Children with Prader-Willi Syndrome."

52. Claudia Ciaccio et al., "Fragile X Syndrome: A Review of Clinical and Molecular Diagnoses," *Italian Journal of Pediatrics* 43, no. 39 (2017): 1–12, https://doi.org/10.1186/s13052-017-0355-y.

53. Chariyawan Charalsawadi et al., "Common Clinical Characteristics and Rare Medical Problems of Fragile X Syndrome in Thai Patients and Review of the Literature," *International Journal of Pediatrics* 2017 (2017): 1–11, https://doi.org/10.1155/2017/9318346.

54. John A. Tsiouris and W. Ted Brown, "Neuropsychiatric Symptoms of Fragile X Syndrome," *CNS Drugs* 18, no. 11 (2004): 687–703, https://doi.org/10.2165/00023210-200418110-00001.

55. Tsiouris and Brown, "Neuropsychiatric Symptoms of Fragile X Syndrome"; Ciaccio et al., "Fragile X Syndrome"; and Charalsawadi et al., "Common Clinical Characteristics and Rare Medical Problems of Fragile X Syndrome in Thai Patients and Review of the Literature."

56. Tsiouris and Brown, "Neuropsychiatric Symptoms of Fragile X Syndrome."

57. Tsiouris and Brown, "Neuropsychiatric Symptoms of Fragile X Syndrome."

58. Ciaccio et al., "Fragile X Syndrome."

59. A. C. Wheeler et al., "Aggression in Fragile X Syndrome," *Journal of Intellectual Disability Research* 60, no. 2 (2016): 113–125, https://doi.org/10.1111/jir.12238.

60. Peter Camfield and Carol Camfield, "Incidence, Prevalence, and Aetiology of Seizures and Epilepsy in Children," *Epileptic Disorders* 17, no. 2 (2015): 117–123, https://doi/10.1684/epd.2015.0736.

61. Elizabeth Berry-Kravis et al., "Seizures in Fragile X Syndrome: Characteristics and Comorbid Diagnoses," *American Journal on Intellectual and Developmental Disabilities* 115, no. 6 (2010): 461–472, https://doi.org/10.1352/1944-7558-115.6.461.

62. Magali Gauthey et al., "Status Epilepticus in Fragile X Syndrome," *Epilepsia* 51, no. 12 (2010): 2,470–2,473, https://doi.org/10.1111/j.1528-1167.2010.02761.x.

63. Sanjay P. Singh, Shubhi Agarwal, and M. Faulkner, "Refractory Status Epilepticus," *Annals of Indian Academy of Neurology* 17, sup. S1 (2014): 32–36, https://doi.org/10.4103/0972-2327.128647.

64. Singh, Agarwal, and Faulkner, "Refractory Status Epilepticus."

65. N. Dörrie et al., "Fetal Alcohol Spectrum Disorders," *European Child & Adolescent Psychiatry* 23, no. 10 (2014): 863–875, https://doi.org/10.1007/s00787-014-0571-6.

66. Dörrie et al., "Fetal Alcohol Spectrum Disorders."

67. Abdelmageed Abdelrahman and Richard Conn, "Eye Abnormalities in Fetal Alcohol Syndrome," *Ulster Medical Journal* 78, no. 3 (2009): 164–165; Dörrie et al., "Fetal Alcohol Spectrum Disorders"; Nguyen X. Thanh and Egon Jonsson, "Life Expectancy of People with Fetal Alcohol Syndrome," *Journal of Population Therapeutics and Clinical Pharmacology* 23, no. 1 (2016): E53–E59; Jenny Rangmar et al., "Cognitive and Executive Functions, Social Cognition and Sense of Coherence in Adults with Fetal Alcohol Syndrome," *Nordic Journal of Psychiatry* 69, no. 6 (2015): 472–478, https://doi.org/10.3109/08039488.2015.1009487; Nadine M. Lindinger et al., "Theory of Mind in Children with Fetal Alcohol Spectrum Disorders," *Alcoholism: Clinical and Experimental Research* 40, no. 2 (2016): 367–376, https://doi.org/10.1111/acer.12961; Danielle Kingdon, Christopher Cardoso, and Jennifer J. McGrath, "Research Review: Executive Function Deficits in Fetal Alcohol Spectrum Disorders and Attention-Deficit/

Hyperactivity Disorder—A Meta-Analysis," *Journal of Child Psychology and Psychiatry* 57, no. 2 (2015): 116–131, https://doi.org/10.1111/jcpp.12451; and H. Eugene Hoyme et al., "Updated Clinical Guidelines for Diagnosing Fetal Alcohol Spectrum Disorders," *Pediatrics* 138, no. 2 (2016): 1–18.

68. Amor-Salamanca and Menchon, "Pain Underreporting Associated with Profound Intellectual Disability in Emergency Departments."

4

Hearing, Vision, and Speech Impairments

Deaf and Hard of Hearing

Tones drop for a five-year-old girl, bitten by a dog. You arrive on scene and her hysterical mother rushes toward you with her daughter, Emily, in her arms. She tells you they had been visiting neighbors when Emily, who had been playing with the dog, was bitten in the face. You do a quick assessment and see the child's right eye is swollen shut, with puncture wounds above and below the orbit. As you attempt to get the mother to give you the child so you can assess and treat, she refuses to step back, saying her daughter is deaf and she needs to be able to communicate with her using American Sign Language. Due to the severity of the injury, and its location, you request aeromedical transport to the nearest pediatric facility. While you wait for the helicopter to arrive, the mother tells you that although Emily had been playing appropriately with the dog, because she could not hear, she missed the growls and low barks from the dog signaling that he was unhappy.

Hearing loss is not uncommon. Fifteen percent of adults in the United States report they have some difficulty hearing, ranging from a slight loss to complete deafness.[1] Congenital hearing loss (present at birth) is seen in 2 to 3 babies per 1,000 live births.[2] According to Gallaudet University,[3] an institute for higher education for those who are deaf and hard of hearing, 9 to 22 out of 1,000 people identify as having a severe hearing loss or are deaf.[4]

Ear anatomy

The ear is divided into three sections: outer, middle, and inner. The *outer ear* consists of the external ear and the ear canal. Sound waves enter the external ear and travel down the ear canal to the middle ear (fig. 4–1).

The *middle ear* starts at the tympanic membrane, or eardrum, and includes the three small bones (*ossicles*) and the eustachian tube, which connects the middle ear to the nasopharynx.[5] Sound waves continue through the middle ear and are transmitted to the inner ear via the ossicles.

The *inner ear* consists of the cochlea, which is the organ of hearing, the semicircular canals that are responsible for balance, and the auditory nerve (cranial nerve VIII), which transmits sounds to the brain for processing.

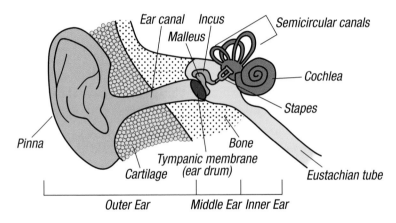

Fig. 4–1. Ear anatomy is divided into three sections.

Types of hearing loss/deafness

A *conductive hearing loss* happens when the sound waves are unable to be conducted, or moved, through the outer and/or middle ear.[6] A *sensorineural hearing loss* occurs when there is damage or deformity in the cochlea or to the nerves that run from the inner ear to the brain.[7] A *mixed hearing loss* means that both conductive and sensorineural losses are present.

Causes of hearing loss/deafness

Hearing loss can occur for a variety of reasons, including genetics, illness, injury, and aging (see table 4–1).

Table 4–1. Common reasons for hearing loss by type of loss

Causes of Hearing Loss by Type	
Conductive	**Sensorineural**
• Fluid buildup in the middle ear	• Genetics
• Otitis media (middle ear infection)	• Osteoporosis
• Otitis externa (outer ear infection or "swimmer's ear")	• Infections (measles, meningitis, malaria, etc.)
• Eustachian tube dysfunction	• Noise
• Damaged tympanic membrane	• Head trauma
• Blockage of the ear canal from wax or foreign object	• Ototoxic drugs (including some antibiotics, chemotherapy drugs, loop diuretics, and aspirin)
• Tumors in the ear canal	
• Deformities in the structure of the outer or middle ear	• Tumors
	• Aging
	• Sickle cell disease

Sources: Hain, "Hearing Loss: An Overview"; American Speech-Language-Hearing Association, "Conductive Hearing Loss"; O. K. Kahveci et al., "Patients with Osteoporosis Have Higher Incidence of Sensorineural Hearing Loss," *Clinical Otolaryngology* 39, no. 3 (2014): 145–149; Sizheng S. Zhao and Ian J. Mackenzie, "Deafness: Malaria as a Forgotten Cause," *Annals of Tropical Paediatrics* 31, no. 1 (2011): 1–10, https://doi.org/10.1179/1465328 11x12925735813724; John C. Carey and Janice C. Palumbos, "Advances in the Understanding of the Genetic Causes of Hearing Loss in Children Inform a Rational Approach to Evaluation," *The Indian Journal of Pediatrics* 83, no. 10 (2016): 1,150–1,156, https://doi. org/10.1007/s12098-015-1941-x; Vishakha W. Rawool and Lynda A. Colligon-Wayne, "Auditory Lifestyles and Beliefs Related to Hearing Loss among College Students in the USA," *Noise and Health* 10, no. 38 (2008): 1–10, https://doi.org/10.4103/1463-1741.39002; Musa T. Samdi et al., "Risk Factors and Identifiable Causes of Hearing Impairment among Pediatric Age Group in Kaduna, Nigeria," *Indian Journal of Otology* 23, no. 4 (2017): 241–243, https://doi.org/10.4103/indianjotol.indianjotol_68_17; Walter E. Nance, "The Genetics of Deafness," *Mental Retardation and Developmental Disabilities Research Reviews* 9, no. 2 (2003): 109–119, https://doi.org/10.1002/mrdd.10067; Austin S. Rose et al., "Noise Exposure Levels in Stock Car Auto Racing," *Ear, Nose & Throat Journal* 87, no. 12 (2008): 689–692; Shubhankur Gupta, Anil Pandey, and Rahul, "Audiometric Analysis of Different Causes of Hearing Loss in Patients Attending a Tertiary Level Hospital in India," *International Archives of Integrated Medicine*, 3, no. 10 (2016): 1–6; Pamela A. Mudd, "Ototoxicity," Medscape.com, 2016.

Remediation

Many people who are deaf do not consider their deafness a disability or limitation. They communicate primarily through sign language and do not use hearing aids or cochlear implants. Others, however, choose to attempt to restore some or all of their hearing through hearing aids or cochlear implants.

- Hearing aids pick up and amplify sound, using a microphone, amplifier, and speaker. They can be worn behind the ear, in the external ear, or inside the ear canal and are most helpful for people with a sensorineural loss.[8]
- Cochlear implants are a more complex hearing restoration option, requiring surgical implantation. Instead of amplifying sound, a cochlear implant bypasses the damaged part of the ear and directly stimulates the auditory nerve. A cochlear implant has both internal (the receiver and electrodes) and external (speech processor) components. The external components are attached to the individual's head via an implanted magnet.[9]

Communicating with people who are deaf/hard-of-hearing

- Sign language, including American Sign Language and Signed Exact English (either directly or through an interpreter)
- Written communication (on paper or electronically via texting or another platform)
- Lip/speech reading (not very effective)

Suggestions for more effective communication

- Remember that not every deaf/hard-of-hearing person can lip read or hear you even with a hearing aid or cochlear implant.
- Gain the person's attention with a hand wave or gentle touch.
- Remember to face the person as you speak to them. Do not turn away to look at your monitor or other equipment while you are speaking.
- Use gestures and facial expressions to help convey meaning.
- Do not exaggerate when speaking but do speak slowly and clearly.
- Do not cover your mouth or speak with gum in your mouth.
- Consider writing on paper or texting to communicate.
- If using an interpreter (family member or professional) speak directly to the patient rather than to the interpreter.

Implications for EMS

- Hearing aids and cochlear implants can be easily lost. Watch for and do not lose hearing aids or external parts of cochlear implants, especially after a mechanical force trauma.

- Confirm with the patient that they are comfortable having a family member act as an on-scene interpreter. Do not assume that they are comfortable sharing their medical issues with a family member or friend.

- If an interpreter is needed, radio ahead to the hospital to arrange for an interpreter to be present upon your arrival to the emergency department.

- Reduce background noise (such as sirens) and maintain sufficient interior lighting in the ambulance to allow the patient to be able to see your mouth, gestures, and other communication attempts.

- Consider learning a few signs to help you communicate with deaf or hard-of-hearing patients (fig. 4–2). There are many free websites that show pictures or videos of medically relevant signs. A particularly helpful site is https://www.medicalasl.com/.

Speech Impairments

You are assessing a 21-year-old male with a chief complaint of abdominal pain. As you ask Jake questions, you notice that he is having difficulty getting the words out. As he speaks, you notice that he is doing a lot of blinking and turning his head. You ask if he is having eye pain or difficulty seeing, which only makes him more frustrated. Jake's mother, Ann, arrives on scene. She tells you that Jake has always had a significant stutter that gets worse in high-stress situations. She also explains that the eye blinking and head movements are strategies he uses to try to speak more fluently. Ann suggests that you speak to Jake as you would with anyone, as he gets more frustrated and finds it harder to speak when he thinks people are impatient with him and his speech. Armed with this helpful information, you return to your assessment and transport Jake to the emergency department.

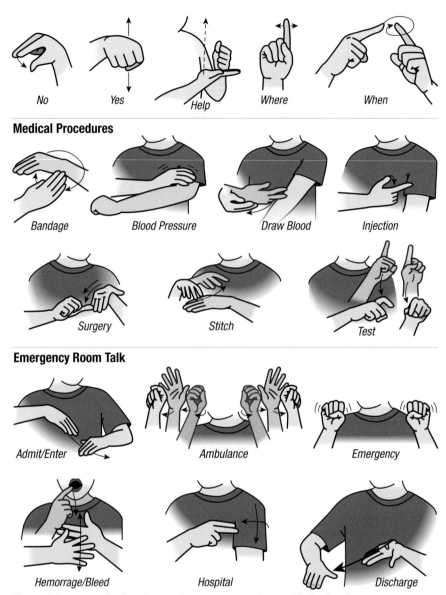

No   Yes   Help   Where   When

Medical Procedures

Bandage   Blood Pressure   Draw Blood   Injection

Surgery   Stitch   Test

Emergency Room Talk

Admit/Enter   Ambulance   Emergency

Hemorrage/Bleed   Hospital   Discharge

Fig. 4–2. Learn medically relevant signs to communicate with deaf patients.
Courtesy: WPClipart, https://www.wpclipart.com/sign_language/ASL_words/index.html.

Speech impairments can make it difficult to understand the individual when they are speaking, which can have a significant impact on an EMS assessment. Speech impairments in children and adults can result from many causes, including strokes, traumatic brain injuries, cleft lip/palate, Parkinson's disease, childhood or acquired apraxia, deafness/hard of hearing, and others.

By themselves the speech disorders will not result in the need for an EMS response, but their presence can cause challenges during assessment and treatment. You may have great difficulty understanding the patients, and they also may have difficulty expressing themselves by speaking.

Apraxia

Apraxia is a neurological disorder in which neuromuscular deficits impair the precision of speech.[10] The individual with apraxia has difficulty with the motor planning required for speaking. It can be caused by brain tumors, strokes, and pregnancy or birth trauma. Apraxia can be comorbid with autism spectrum disorders or other behavior-related disorders, or it may have no known cause.

The American Speech-Language-Hearing Association describes several characteristics of apraxic speech:

- Vowel and consonant distortions
- Vowel, consonant, and syllable omissions
- Addition of the schwa sound (uh) into words
- Differences in prosody (rate, pitch, and loudness)
- Loss of words or sounds
- Transposing sounds in words ("batel" for "table")

Children with apraxia of speech can also have additional gross and fine motor delays and difficulties.

Articulation impairments

Articulation refers to the production of speech sounds. Impairments in articulation can manifest in a variety of ways.[11] Dialect variations or accents in speech should not be confused with disordered speech. Articulation errors can be very mild, only impacting one or two sounds, or they can be very severe, with the individual being extremely hard to understand.

Types of articulation errors, in order of decreasing severity of impact on understanding, include the following:

- Omissions of sounds
  - "ook" for "book"
  - "ca" for "cat"
  - "tuck" for "truck"

- Substitutions of sounds
  - "wain" for "rain"
  - "fum" for "thumb"
- Additions of sounds
  - "ar-uh" for "are"
- Distortions of sounds
  - The sounds are present but unclear. Common with r, s, and l.

In addition to their impact on intelligibility of speech, articulation errors can also have a negative impact on children's self-esteem, confidence, and academic learning.

Fluency disorders

Fluent speech is smooth and effortless.[12] All of us can have moments when we trip up on what we are trying to say or get a little "tongue-tied," but true speech *disfluencies* (more commonly known as "stuttering" and "cluttering") can have a significant impact on an individual's ability to communicate. This in turn can affect their self-esteem and cause fear and embarrassment related to speaking.

There are many theories on the causes of disfluencies, but the most common causes are thought to be gene mutations and structural and functional differences in the brain. It is not *caused* by emotional or psychological problems but can certainly *result* in those issues. Disfluencies can also be temporarily exacerbated by stressful situations, such as a medical or traumatic emergency with themselves or a loved one.

Stuttering

Stuttering is the repetition, hesitation, or prolongation of sounds or words. The individual may repeat the beginning sound in a word or the entire word. They may hesitate or become blocked when trying to speak, not able to get the word out, or they may prolong or extend sounds in words.

- *Repetition.* "I want to pet the c-c-c-c-cat," or "I-I-I-I want to pet the cat."
- *Hesitation.* "I want to p-----------et the cat," or "I want to ---------pet the cat."
- *Prolongation.* "I want to pet the caaaaaaaaaaaat."

In addition to these speech challenges, people who stutter may also have secondary behaviors that are acquired/learned behaviors that appear in an attempt to prevent or stop a stuttering moment. These can vary widely but include extra sounds, eye blinking, facial/head movements, leg tapping or shaking, and fist clenching, and can be interfering and distracting in their own way. You may also notice a great deal of physical struggle as they speak.

Cluttering

Cluttering is characterized by speech that can be rapid at times, with irregular pacing or pausing, along with the running together of words and/or deletions of syllables, causing difficulty with being understood by the listener. Cluttering can occur in conjunction with other disorders such as ADHD, learning disabilities, and autism spectrum disorders. It can be very difficult to understand some individuals who clutter, especially on the phone.

Implications for EMS

- Do not finish their sentences for them or try to anticipate what they are going to say.
- If you do not understand them, let them know. They may be able to communicate with you in another way (gestures, writing, pointing, etc.).
- Limit your questions to one at a time, waiting for their response.
- You may find that the more you listen to them, the easier it is for you to understand them.
- Speak directly to them, not their caregiver.
- Be prepared for an assistive communication device. Allow them to use it during assessment and be sure to bring it with you in the ambulance.
- If they are using a communication device, remember that it is their voice. Allow them to finish typing, do not assume or guess what they are trying to say, and do not read over their shoulder.
- Communicating with people who stutter can be anxiety producing or frustrating for the listener. When talking with someone who stutters, consider the following suggestions:

- Talk to them normally. You do not need to raise your voice or speak slowly. They can understand you. Speak as you would to anyone else.
- Keep natural eye contact.
- Relax, but don't tell them to relax. Also, don't tell them to slow down or take a deep breath. They know best how to manage their stutter.
- Listen and pay attention to the words, not the delivery.
- Don't interrupt.

Vision Impairments

You are dispatched for injuries from a fall for a 58-year-old female. Upon your arrival, you hear your patient, Charlotte, calling you from inside the residence saying that the door is open and the dog near her will not hurt you. You find Charlotte sitting on the floor with her guide dog, Frank, sitting close and protectively. Charlotte has Frank under voice control as he is not wearing his harness, which is typical when they are home. Charlotte states she is blind but can see some lights and shadows. She had repair people in to do some work and they moved the furniture without putting it back when they left. Not knowing it was there, she tripped and twisted her knee and is unable to get up. You splint Charlotte's knee while your partner goes to get Frank's harness from Charlotte's bedroom at her direction. At this point, Charlotte's husband, Steve, arrives home. Although you are prepared to take Frank with you in the ambulance, Steve says he will bring Frank with him to the emergency department so he can be safely secured in his vehicle. You help Charlotte to the stretcher, support her knee with pillows underneath, and depart for the hospital, where she will reunite with Frank.

The World Health Organization estimates that 253 million people worldwide have varying degrees of vision impairment, ranging from moderate vision loss to complete blindness.[13] Fifty million people worldwide are reported to be totally blind, with 80% of those cases being in people over the age of 50.[14] According to the Centers for Disease Control and Prevention, "Twenty-one million Americans report functional vision problems or eye conditions that may compromise vision," with risk increasing with age.[15]

Many people who are considered blind have some residual vision and may be able to see some light, shapes, or colors. Legal blindness was defined by the US government in 1935 as follows:[16]

- *Visual acuity* (how clearly one sees something) of 20/200 or worse *with corrective lenses.*

- *Visual field* (what one can see in the periphery) of 20° or less. A typical visual field is 160° horizontally and 110° vertically.[17]

The National Eye Institute, a section of the National Institutes of Health, describes more than 30 different types of eye conditions that can contribute to vision loss or blindness.[18] Some of the more common disorders are described below.

- *Amblyopia*, also called "lazy eye," is a condition in which one eye has significantly poorer vision than the other eye. This can be caused by muscle misalignment (strabismus; see below). Amblyopia is treated through glasses or patching of the strong eye to encourage the weak eye. If the cause is muscle misalignment, surgical correction may be an option. Amblyopia can cause problems with depth perception, as people need both eyes working together to perceive depth and distance.

- *Blepharitis* is an inflammation of the inner or outer eyelids that can lead to a *sty* (infection of the oil glands), a *chalazion* (inflammation of the oil glands), or disruptions in tear production causing increased tearing or dry eyes.

- *Cataracts* are a clouding of the lens located behind the iris and pupil. They are caused when the proteins in the lens stick together and limit the amount of light that can pass through the eye. Cataracts are extremely common in the elderly (especially those over 80 years of age). They rarely occur in children and are usually due to genetics or pregnancy complications, such as an infection.[19] Smoking and diabetes can also increase the risk. Glasses can help reduce some of the effects of cataracts, but the only way to restore vision is through surgery to replace the cloudy lens with an artificial lens.

- *Glaucoma* is an eye disease characterized by an increase in the pressure inside the eye that results in damage to the optic nerve and retina. Progression of the disease leads to a gradual loss of the peripheral vision or visual field. Glaucoma can be treated with medication (drops or pills) or surgery, but lost vision cannot be regained.

- *Macular degeneration* is the deterioration of the macula (the center of the retina). Macular degeneration results in loss of central vision, while peripheral vision remains undamaged. The risk for macular degeneration increases with genetic tendencies, age, and smoking.

- *Retinal detachment* occurs when the light-sensitive tissue of the retina that is responsible for sending visual messages to the optic nerve separates or detaches from the back of the eye. If the retina detaches from the back of the eye, it can cause permanent vision loss. The retina can detach with retinal inflammation, eye injury, if a retinal tear worsens, or rarely, if scar tissue pulls the retina. Symptoms of a retinal detachment include an increase in floaters or floating specks, along with vivid flashes of light. Because a retinal detachment can cause permanent vision loss, this is a medical emergency. Treatment can involve laser surgery or freezing for small detachments. Larger detachments are treated with more invasive surgery.

- *Strabismus* is muscle misalignment that results in the eyes turning inward (*esotropia* or "crossed eyes"), outward (*exotropia* or "wall eyes"), upward (*hypertropia*), or downward (*hypotropia*). This is a fairly common disorder in the pediatric population and is often present in children with no other health problems. Children with disorders that affect the brain, however, such as cerebral palsy or hydrocephalus, are at greater risk for strabismus. Pediatric strabismus can linger or recur in adulthood, but adult onset strabismus can be caused by stroke, trauma, or neurological problems and should be taken seriously. Strabismus can cause amblyopia and double vision. Treatment options include glasses, glasses with prism lenses, and muscle realignment surgery.[20]

Implications for EMS

- With the exception of a retinal detachment, these eye conditions in themselves are unlikely to result in an EMS response. Secondary issues can occur, however, especially injuries resulting from not being able to see well or at all.

- Be sure to identify yourself by name and role. If there is more than one provider in the ambulance, reidentify yourself by name when you speak to them.

- Speak directly to the patient, not a caregiver, if you would ordinarily speak to that person if they were sighted.

- If you will be walking with your patient (to another room or to the ambulance), offer your arm or elbow for them to take rather than you taking their arm. When you are helping them to the stretcher, place their hand on the raised head of the stretcher so they can orient to its location.

- Vision loss can occur in varying degrees, so don't assume that a patient who identifies as blind can see nothing.

- Children who are blind or have low vision may be highly tactile. Let them touch things before using them, such as the blood pressure cuff or your stethoscope so they can familiarize themselves with what is going to be touching them. But at the same time, watch for things going into their mouths!

- Provide lots of verbal support and direction. Tell them that you are going to touch them and tell them exactly what you intend to do, especially if you are planning to move them.

- Don't be afraid to use words like "look" and "see." If you actively try to avoid those words, it could become awkward for both of you.

- Be prepared for a guide dog (see chapter 1 for more information on service animals). If they use a white cane, bring it with you during transport.

- When you leave your patient at the hospital, don't forget to tell them you are leaving as they will not be able to see you leave the room. They will need to know that you have transferred their care to the hospital staff.

- Don't shout.
- If your patient is exhibiting signs of strabismus, be sure to inquire if it is a residual pediatric condition or a new onset problem. If the latter, consider acute problems (stroke, trauma, etc.) that could be the cause.
- A retinal detachment is a medical emergency. If you suspect your patient is experiencing a retinal detachment due to a sudden onset or worsening of floaters or light flashes, consider transport to an eye specialty center.

Notes

1. D. L. Blackwell, J. W. Lucas, and T. C. Clarke, *Summary Health Statistics for U.S. Adults: National Health Interview Survey, 2012, DHHS Publication No. 2014–1588*, Series 10, no. 260 (Hyattsville, Maryland: National Center for Health Statistics, CDC, US DHHS, February 2014): 1–171, reprint, https://www.cdc.gov/nchs/data/series/sr_10/sr10_260.pdf.

2. M. Gaffney et al., "Identifying Infants with Hearing Loss—United States, 1999–2007," *Morbidity and Mortality Weekly Report* 59, no. 8 (2010): 1–36, reprint.

3. General information about Gallaudet University may be viewed at https://www.gallaudet.edu/.

4. R. E. Mitchell, "Can You Tell Me How Many Deaf People There Are in the United States?" February 15, 2005, retrieved May 22, 2018, https://research.gallaudet.edu/Demographics/deaf-US.php.

5. Ted L. Tewfik, "Eustachian Tube Function: Overview, Embryology of the Eustachian Tube, Anatomy of the Eustachian Tube," Medscape, May 9, 2018, retrieved May 22, 2018, https://emedicine.medscape.com/article/874348-overview.

6. T. C. Hain, "Hearing Loss: An Overview," American Research Hearing Foundation, October 2012, retrieved May 22, 2018, https://www.american-hearing.org/disease/hearing-loss-an-overview/.

7. Hain, "Hearing Loss."

8. US Department of Health and Human Services, National Institutes of Health, National Institute on Deafness and Other Communication Disorders, "NIDCD Fact Sheet: Hearing and Balance, Hearing Aids," National Institutes of Health, NIH Publication No. 99-4340 (September 2013), https://www.nidcd.nih.gov/sites/default/files/Documents/health/hearing/nidcd-hearing-aids.pdf.

9. US Department of Health and Human Services, National Institutes of Health, National Institute on Deafness and Other Communication Disorders, "NIDCD Fact Sheet: Hearing and Balance, Cochlear Implants," National Institutes of Health, NIH Publication No. 00-4798 (February 2016), https://www.nidcd.nih.gov/sites/default/files/Documents/health/hearing/CochlearImplants.pdf.

10. American Speech-Language-Hearing Association, "Childhood Apraxia of Speech," retrieved April 3, 2018, https://www.asha.org/Practice-Portal/Clinical-Topics/Childhood-Apraxia-of-Speech/; and Alexandra Basilakos et al., "A Multivariate Analytic Approach to the Differential Diagnosis of Apraxia of Speech," *Journal of Speech Language and Hearing Research* 60, no. 12 (2017): 3,378–3,392, https://doi.org/10.1044/2017_jslhr-s-16-0443.

11. Graham R. Daniel and Sharynne Mcleod, "Children with Speech Sound Disorders at School: Challenges for Children, Parents, and Teachers," *Australian Journal of Teacher Education* (2017): 81–101, https://doi.org/10.14221/ajte.2017v42n2.6; American Speech-Language-Hearing Association, "Speech Sound Disorders: Articulation and Phonology," https://www.asha.org/Practice-Portal/Clinical-Topics/Articulation-and-Phonology/.

12. American Speech-Language-Hearing Association, "Childhood Fluency Disorders," retrieved May 22, 2018, https://www.asha.org/Practice-Portal/Clinical-Topics/Childhood-Fluency-Disorders/.

13. World Health Organization, "Blindness and Vision Impairment," October 2017, retrieved May 3, 2018, http://www.who.int/en/news-room/fact-sheets/detail/blindness-and-visual-impairment.

14. Andrew A. Dahl, "Blindness," MedicineNet.com, November 14, 2017, retrieved May 3, 2018, https://www.medicinenet.com/blindness/article.htm#blindness_facts.

15. US Department of Health and Human Services, Centers for Disease Control and Prevention, "The Burden of Vision Loss: Population Estimates," Visual Health Initiative, September 25, 2009, retrieved May 3, 2018, https://www.cdc.gov/visionhealth/basic_information/vision_loss_burden.htm.

16. Dahl, "Blindness."

17. R. H. Spector, "Visual Fields," chap. 116 in *Clinical Methods: The History, Physical, and Laboratory Examinations*, H. K. Walker, W. D. Hall, J. W. Hurst, eds., 3rd ed. (Boston: Butterworth, 1990), https://www.ncbi.nlm.nih.gov/books/NBK220/.

18. WHO, "Blindness and Visual Impairment"; and US Department of Health and Human Services, National Institutes of Health, National Eye Institute, "Learn about Eye Health: Eye Conditions and Diseases—Browse Conditions and Diseases A to Z," retrieved September 17, 2019, https://nei.nih.gov/learn-about-eye-health/eye-conditions-and-diseases.

19. WebMD, "Cataracts in Children: Topic Overview," 2015, retrieved May 3, 2018, https://www.webmd.com/children/tc/cataracts-in-children-topic-overview#1.

20. American Association for Pediatric Ophthalmology and Strabismus, "Strabismus," February 12, 2018, retrieved September 17, 2019, https://aapos.org/browse/glossary/entry?GlossaryKey=f95036af-4a14-4397-bf8f-87e3980398b4.

5

Physical Disabilities

Multiple tones start dropping for a motor vehicle accident with injuries. There are at least two cars involved with possible entrapment. Once on scene, command directs you to your patient in the front passenger seat of a vehicle that is just off the road. Firefighters are still securing the vehicle as you approach. The vehicle has damage to the right front and the airbags were deployed. Your patient, George, is alert and calm. He denies any loss of consciousness and states he remembers everything. Other than some slight neck pain, he denies injury. You place a cervical collar as you obtain initial vitals and continue asking assessment questions. You tell George that you are going to conduct a trauma assessment to look for injury. He agrees to the assessment and says that his legs are paralyzed after a car accident 15 years ago that damaged his lumbar spine and he has no feeling in his legs. Further assessment reveals a stable pelvis but also a deformity in George's right thigh that is indicative of a femur fracture. You send your partner for the traction splint and alert the firefighters that you need to move expeditiously to extricate George from the vehicle onto a long spine board for subsequent transport to a trauma center.

A physical or orthopedic disability is an impairment involving the bones, joints, and muscles and can cause complications with EMS assessment and transport. These impairments can be the result of a prenatal or postnatal injury, a genetic or nongenetic condition, or a disease (table 5–1).

Table 5–1. Types of orthopedic impairments

Types of Orthopedic Impairments		
Genetic Conditions	**Nongenetic Conditions**	**Diseases**
• Ehlers-Danlos syndrome • Cleft lip/palate • Dwarfism • Osteogenesis imperfecta	• Cerebral palsy (may have some genetic component) • Spina bifida • Spinal cord injuries	• Rheumatoid arthritis • Osteoarthritis

Arthritis

Janet is a 48-year-old woman who called 911 for generalized pain all over, as well as a new onset of abdominal pain. When you arrive, she is sitting in her residence, looking unwell. Janet tells you that she has osteoarthritis that is particularly bad in her hands and back. The only medication she reports using is a nonsteroidal anti-inflammatory. She takes it frequently (even admitting to taking more than the recommended amount) with little relief and now is complaining of abdominal pain. While you are assessing her, she vomits dark blood. Janet denies a history of gastrointestinal bleeding. Her vitals remain stable, but she continues to feel severe nausea. After conducting a 12-lead EKG to ensure she does not have a long QTc interval, you insert an IV and administer ondansetron for the nausea. You monitor Janet carefully during transport to the closest emergency department for evaluation.

Rheumatoid arthritis

Rheumatoid arthritis (RA), reported in modern literature for more than a century,[1] is a type of autoimmune inflammatory arthritis that has a typical onset between 30 and 50 years of age.[2] RA affects just under 1% of the worldwide adult population.[3] Juvenile rheumatoid arthritis has an onset in children younger than 16 years,[4] with a prevalence of approximately 113 per 100,000.[5] RA is thought to be triggered by both genetic and environmental factors. It is a progressive disease characterized by periods of flare-ups and remissions.[6]

Rheumatoid arthritis causes joint and *extra-articular* (outside the joint) inflammation that leads to damage and chronic pain.[7] The body's immune system attacks tissues and causes inflammation that leads to decreased range of motion, stiffness, swelling, and deformity. In joints, the synovial tissue becomes inflamed, resulting in damage to ligaments, cartilage, and bone, causing its characteristic joint deformation.[8] Joints affected by rheumatoid arthritis are typically enlarged, deformed, and painful, with redness, swelling, and warmth. Commonly affected joints include bilateral hands, wrists, elbows, knees, shoulders, and neck.[9] Morning stiffness, which can be severe, is also typical and can last more than an hour. Muscle weakness is also common, along with a low-grade fever and fatigue.[10]

Rheumatoid arthritis is a *systemic disease*, meaning the inflammation can impact the entire body.[11]

- *Eyes and mouth.* The tear and salivary glands can become inflamed, leading to dry eyes and mouth. It can cause corneal abrasions, scleritis, dental decay and cavities, mouth sores, and parotid gland stones.
- *Lungs.* Inflammation of the lining of the lungs, or pleuritis, can cause difficulty breathing, chest pain, and coughing.
- *Heart.* Inflammation of the lining of the heart, or pericarditis, can also cause chest pain and an increased risk of heart attack.
- *Lymph nodes.* There is a higher risk of lymphoma in patients with rheumatoid arthritis.
- *Blood vessels.* Vasculitis, or inflammation of the blood vessels, can impede blood circulation and lead to tissue necrosis.

Treatment is typically pharmacological, with acetaminophen and opiates for pain management, oral corticosteroids and nonsteroidal anti-inflammatory drugs (NSAIDs) to reduce inflammation, and disease-modifying antirheumatic drugs (DMARDs) to slow the progression of joint damage.[12]

Osteoarthritis

Osteoarthritis (OA), also called *degenerative joint disease* (*DJD*), is the most common of joint diseases and affects more than 30 million people in the US.[13] OA is thought to be caused by multiple factors, including heredity, as part of the natural aging process, and sometimes secondary to disease (e.g., gout, avascular necrosis), injury (e.g., broken ankle, sprained knee), and/or frequent repetitive movements of a joint (e.g., typing, throwing a football). It is not an autoimmune process nor a systemic disease.[14]

OA shares many of the characteristics of RA, but it is degenerative in nature rather than inflammatory. Unlike RA, which usually causes damage to symmetrical joints (e.g., both elbows and knees) and joint deformation, OA does not typically affect symmetric joints (e.g., just the left elbow and the right knee) and does not cause joint deformity.[15] In osteoarthritis, the cartilage that cushions and protects a joint degenerates, eventually resulting in bone on bone movement and friction, which limits the joint mobility and causes pain. This promotes the growth of *osteophytes*, also called "bone spurs," which further limit movement. This process causes pain, decreased range of motion, swelling, and stiffness. Because osteoarthritis is not a systemic disease, the pain and inflammation is limited to the affected joints. Note that in RA the inflammation causes the damage to tissues, while in OA inflammation is the result of joint damage. OA commonly affects the hands, feet, spine, and large weight-bearing joints like the hips and knees.[16]

Treatment for OA includes nonpharmaceutical methods such as losing weight if obese, avoiding activities that stress the affected joints, ice and heat compresses, physical therapy for affected joints, and devices like knee braces and lumbar support belts. Pharmaceutical methods include pain medications, oral and injected NSAIDs, and injected corticosteroids and hyaluronic acid to reduce inflammation. Surgical methods include arthroscopies and joint replacements (fig. 5–1).[17]

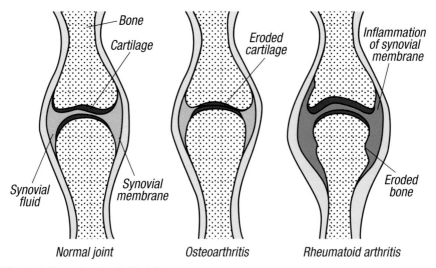

Fig. 5–1. Normal and arthritic joints

Implications for EMS

- Consider pain management.
- Treat secondary signs and symptoms from systemic problems as appropriate.
- Regular use of NSAIDs can cause stomach upset and pain, as well as diarrhea and possible gastrointestinal bleeding.[18]
- Patients prescribed opioids for pain are at risk for constipation with regular use, as well as dependency, addiction, and overdose with misuse.[19]

Cerebral Palsy

You are en route for a generalized sick call for a 37-year-old male, and no other details are available. Once on scene, you are directed to your patient, Michael, in the residence with his parents present. Michael's parents tell you that he has cerebral palsy, cannot walk, and speaks with great difficulty. They tell you he is complaining of not feeling well and appears a little sluggish. You approach Michael, who is sitting in his wheelchair, and start to ask assessment questions, but as his parents told you, he is very hard to understand. While you continue to direct your questions to Michael, you also look to his parents for help in understanding, which they provide. You ascertain that he generally feels unwell. You work toward obtaining vital signs, which is difficult to do because his limbs are contracted and do not straighten or move easily. Because Michael cannot move on his own, you ask him and his parents for suggestions on how to move him safely and comfortably from his wheelchair to the stretcher. Once on the stretcher, you make sure that his limbs are well supported and that all the voids are padded. Michael's parents will meet you at the hospital and will bring his wheelchair with them.

Cerebral palsy is an umbrella term that describes a group of signs and symptoms related to motor abnormalities caused by damage to the brain during fetal development or in the neonatal period. This damage can have different causes that include abnormal brain development, decreased oxygenation to the brain (before, during, or after birth), prematurity and associated complications, infection, and cerebral hemorrhage.[20] Individuals with cerebral palsy can have a variety of symptoms, ranging from very mild to very severe. The condition is nonprogressive, meaning the severity typically does not worsen over time, although the clinical presentation may change as a person's nervous system matures.[21]

The most common type of cerebral palsy is *spastic cerebral palsy*, representing 80% to 90% of cases. Spastic cerebral palsy is characterized by an increase in muscle tone resulting in varying degrees of paralysis, increased reflexes, tightness, and stiffness of muscles. This type of cerebral palsy can be *hemiplegic* (involving one side of the body), *diplegic* (affecting both lower extremities), or *quadriplegic* (affecting all four extremities and the torso).[22]

Dyskinetic cerebral palsy accounts for 10% to 15% of cases and is characterized by increased muscle tone accompanied by involuntary, abnormal movements. *Ataxic cerebral palsy* comprises less than 5% of cerebral palsy and is characterized by decreased muscle tone and tremors. The remaining cases can be attributed to *mixed cerebral palsy* (a combination of spastic and dyskinetic) and other very uncommon forms.[23]

People with cerebral palsy can have characteristics and complications that may present special challenges for EMS providers. There are issues that are part of cerebral palsy but present similarly to other disabilities. Many people with cerebral palsy have difficulty with movement and walking, and they may have similar complications as described in the section on spina bifida, such as paralysis, skin breakdown, and increased risk of fracture or injury. Up to 60% of people with cerebral palsy have a seizure disorder. Pain is very common, impacting as many as 70% of individuals.[24] Intellectual disability is present in 30% to 50% of people with cerebral palsy.[25] Communication challenges (described in the following text) can make assessing for pain and deciding appropriate pain management difficult. (See the section about pain in chapter 3 on intellectual disabilities.)

There are some issues, however, that are unique to cerebral palsy, and EMS providers should take note of these.

Feeding and swallowing

Because oral motor control can be impacted in cerebral palsy, feeding and swallowing can be problematic. This can lead to an increased risk of choking, failure to thrive/malnourishment, and aspiration pneumonia.[26] In addition to possibly being called for complications related to feeding/swallowing, the

EMS provider will want to be cautious when administering oral medications in order to avoid causing or exacerbating a problem.

Communication

Along with poor oral motor control, people with cerebral palsy can have difficulties with the muscles associated with speaking. This can make speaking difficult, and it can impact the overall intelligibility of speech, making some people with cerebral palsy hard to understand. This is also known as *dysarthria*.[27] Hustad et al. report that children with cerebral palsy are at a significant risk of speech and language delays. They note that although some will outgrow those delays, "Most children with [cerebral palsy] who have early communication problems will have long standing and persistent problems with communication as they mature."[28]

The presentation of speech and voice can vary based on the severity and type of cerebral palsy, as well as with the age of the individual. Some ways that speech and voice can be impacted include the following:[29]

- Frequent *inspirations* (inhalations)
- Fluctuations in pitch and loudness
- Imprecise/impaired articulation (how individual sounds are made)
- Hypernasality (increased airflow through the nose rather than the mouth when speaking)
- Inappropriate pauses
- Slowness
- Breathiness
- Unusual *prosody* (stress and intonation)

Hemsley et al. discussed barriers to communication for people, especially children, with cerebral palsy who were hospitalized.[30] Many of these barriers can be associated with prehospital experiences as well. Some of these barriers include the following:

- *Unfamiliarity with or lack of access to communication devices.* If the individual uses a communication device and it is not available (e.g., it is damaged in an accident or the person's caregiver fails to make it available for hospital transport), then communication will be hindered. If the patient's communication device is available, the parents and/or caregiver usually will be a good source of information on how to use it. Occasionally, however, you might pick up a child from school and the parents are not present or will meet you at the hospital. While the school will send an adult to act *in loco parentis*, it may be an adult who does not know the child well and is unfamiliar with the child's equipment. (For more information, see the section that follows on communication devices.)

- *Lack of time to communicate.* In an emergency situation, time is often of the essence. People with cerebral palsy may be able to speak but may do so slowly or with difficulty, and they can be difficult to understand. This can be frustrating for both the patient and EMS provider and can potentially lead to disastrous miscommunication.

- *Not speaking directly to the patient.* If the patient is having difficulty speaking or otherwise communicating, it is still important to speak directly to them, even when a caregiver is present. Not doing so may be perceived as disrespectful and can limit the building of trust and rapport. If you are unable to understand the speech of a patient with cerebral palsy, their caregiver or family members usually will be able to understand due to their increased familiarity with the patient's speech patterns. Remember to speak directly to your patient and to listen to their responses, but also be prepared for a family member or caregiver to help you with understanding.

- *Not listening to the family or caregiver.* While your patient is your priority and direct communication with them is vital, sometimes it is not always practical or possible. As noted above, another person might need to be their "voice," especially in an emergency situation when things are happening quickly, and lives are potentially at stake. It is also important to remember the feelings and experiences of the family members/caregivers and that they may have important information relevant to the current situation and previous hospitalizations. People with cerebral palsy may need to be hospitalized frequently, depending on the severity of their symptoms. Family members, especially parents of children with cerebral palsy, are often with that person day in and day out, meeting their medical needs. According to a study by Hemsley et al.,[31] these individuals act on behalf of the person with cerebral palsy as "devoted carers,"[32] advocates, and often literally or figuratively as their voice. While you should never let a family member take over your scene, direct care, or ask you to act outside your protocols, it could potentially be a serious mistake to ignore their knowledge and input.

Hemsley et al. collected suggestions from parents of children with cerebral palsy to help hospital staff improve communication with pediatric patients with CP.[33] The resulting suggestions from the parents can also be considered for prehospital settings and for all ages:[34]

- *Be willing to attempt communication.* This is important even if communication is awkward or not completely successful. The parents wanted to remind health care providers that even if the child could not express themselves clearly, they often could understand what was being said to them.

- *Use age-appropriate language.* Treat children like children and adults like adults, even if they are having difficulty communicating.

- *Recognize that communication and understanding might take more time.*

- *Be observant and understand that not all communication is verbal.* You may pick up on nonverbal cues that indicate pain or discomfort. See the section on pain assessment in the chapter on intellectual disabilities.

- *Use communication devices if they are available.* Don't be afraid of technology.

Communication devices

Your patient with cerebral palsy who has associated movement and speech challenges may have an *alternative or augmentative communication (AAC)* device. This can be high-technology like a computerized device that has voice output (including tablets and cell phones), or low-technology like a picture- or word-based board or book where the person points to the pictures or words they wish to use.

The American Speech-Language-Hearing Association[35] defines alternative or augmentative communication as any form of communication other than oral speech. This can include facial expressions, gestures, sign language, pictures, writing, or technology. Augmentative communication helps *support* a person's existing oral language, which may be limited in scope or intelligibility. Alternative communication replaces speech that is absent or unintelligible.

If your patient uses an AAC device, be sure to use it during assessment and bring it along during transport. Not only will you need it in the ambulance, the patient and family/caregivers will also need it while they are in the emergency department and if the patient is admitted. Remember that if your patient does not have their communication support, they do not have a voice. If you deny them access to their device (either intentionally or unintentionally), you are denying them their voice.

Vision problems

People with cerebral palsy have an increased risk of vision problems, including problems with visual field and ocular alignment.[36] This can lead to increased risk of injury, especially for those who are ambulatory.

Gastrointestinal problems

Gastroesophageal reflux and constipation are commonly associated with cerebral palsy.[37] These conditions can cause pain and discomfort and may necessitate visits to the emergency department for management.

Respiratory problems

The musculoskeletal problems associated with cerebral palsy, including muscle contractures and muscle shortening, can lead to *scoliosis* (spine curvature), which in turn can lead to increased difficulty in breathing. This can contribute to pneumonia and respiratory compromise.[38]

Chronic pain

Most people with cerebral palsy, including children, have chronic pain. Cerebral palsy can cause deficits in *somatosensation*, or how the body interprets and responds to touch. This may result in pain, reduced touch sensitivity, *stereognosis* (difficulty identifying items by touch alone), and poor *proprioception* (the awareness and control of one's body position and control over muscle movements and strength).[39]

Implications for EMS

- Do not force limbs to bend or straighten. Work around the person's natural positioning and place them in a position of comfort (even if it doesn't look comfortable to you). Follow their lead on moving and positioning. Ask them what is comfortable.

- You may have difficulty obtaining vital signs in patients who have limb contractures or tremors, especially when using a cardiac monitor. Consider obtaining vital signs manually.
- Be cautious when positioning the patient on the stretcher or stair chair. Pad all the voids and watch for oddly positioned limbs or posture that the patient might not be able to feel or tell you about.
- Remember that the patient may have diminished touch recognition so be especially attentive with trauma assessments.
- Take the patient's mobility equipment with you in the ambulance if at all possible.
- Be prepared for seizures.
- Remember that physical impairments are not necessarily correlated to cognitive competence. The inability to speak, or difficulty speaking, does not mean that the person cannot understand or communicate with you.

Cleft Lip and Palate

You are dispatched for an eight-month-old male who is "not acting right." Upon arrival at the residence you are greeted by the baby's parents, who tell you that their son, Oliver, has not been feeding well for several days and they are having trouble rousing him. As you start to assess Oliver, you see that he has a repaired cleft lip. His parents tell you that he will be undergoing a second repair of his cleft palate in a couple of months. Oliver is sleepy but cries when you tap the soles of his feet. Lung sounds reveal slight wheezing, and Oliver coughs weakly. Because of his cleft palate and reports of feeding difficulties, coupled with your assessment findings, you suspect aspiration of his bottle contents and possible pneumonia. You prepare to transport Oliver to the nearest pediatric facility.

A *cleft lip and palate* occurs during fetal development when the upper lip or palate does not close together, leaving a split, or "cleft" in the hard or soft palate and/or the upper lip. In more severe cases, the cleft lip can extend into the nose and can be unilateral or bilateral. A cleft palate leaves an opening from the hard palate, or roof of the mouth, into the nasopharynx.[40] In some cases, however, the skin that covers the palate is intact, but the structure beneath it is open.[41]

According to the Centers for Disease Control, an estimated 4,440 babies are born each year with a cleft lip (with or without a cleft palate), and 2,650 babies are born with a cleft palate in the United States.[42] Causes of cleft lip/palate vary and include several genetic syndromes (e.g., Pierre Robin syndrome and Treacher Collins syndrome) and those with a family history of cleft lip/palate. Prenatal exposure to alcohol, tobacco, and other drugs increases the risk of cleft lip and palate.[43]

Both cleft lip and cleft palate are treated surgically. The American Cleft Palate-Craniofacial Association recommends that the initial surgery for cleft lip repair, including nasal repair, occur before the child's first birthday and earlier if appropriate.[44] Cleft palate repairs are typically more complicated, resulting in multiple surgeries over multiple years, with the initial palate repair occurring by 18 months of age.

Problems associated with cleft lip and palate

- *Feeding and swallowing.* Very often babies with cleft lip/palates that have not yet been repaired have difficulty feeding, as they have trouble maintaining seal and adequate suction at the breast or bottle. Feeding takes longer, and babies tire easily from the effort. They may fall asleep while feeding and have to feed more frequently in order to gain weight adequately. Milk or formula can go up the nose, and babies can swallow too much air, which can cause abdominal pain, gagging, choking, vomiting, oxygen desaturation, and increased respiratory rate.[45]

- *Dental concerns.* Children with both a cleft lip and a cleft palate have a higher incidence of dental abnormalities, resulting in a greater risk for periodontal disease and the need for orthodontia.

- *Ear infections.* Children with cleft palate are at a greater risk for ear infections and hearing loss, which may result in the surgical insertion of ear tubes, frequent use of antibiotics, and the need for hearing aids.[46] The increased risk of ear infections persists even after surgical repair of the cleft palate due to impaired functioning of the muscles that support the eustachian tube.[47]

- *Sleep apnea.* In some cases, children with cleft lip/palate have an increased risk of sleep apnea due to associated problems with the muscles of the tongue.[48]

- *Speaking.* Due to the role of the hard and soft palate in producing speech, children with cleft palate have difficulty producing some sounds.[49]

Implications for EMS

- Babies, especially before surgical repair, may be at greater risk for aspiration during feeding.
- Babies who do not feed well can quickly become dehydrated or malnourished and subsequently may become lethargic.
- Ear and dental infections can cause fever and pain.
- Attention must be paid to airway management. When manually ventilating infants with an uncorrected cleft lip/palate, be especially careful to maintain a tight seal around the nose and mouth.
- There are additional considerations with endotracheal tube placement during respiratory or cardiac arrest:
  - Laryngoscopy and subsequent intubation in an infant with an unrepaired cleft palate will present additional hurdles to the already challenging pediatric intubation. The deformities present with a cleft palate may interfere with the placement of the laryngoscope and views of the anatomy.[50]
  - Xue et al. provide the following suggestions to facilitate the intubation of an infant with a cleft palate:[51]
    - Place the infant in the sniffing position and pad under the shoulders.
    - Use external laryngeal compression to improve the internal view.
    - Use a pediatric stylet to maintain the shape of the endotracheal tube during insertion.
    - Bend the distal end of the endotracheal tube to a 70° to 80° angle.
    - The authors also emphasize the importance of minimizing repeated intubation attempts and maintaining adequate ventilation through other measures to avoid hypoxia.

Dwarfism

You are dispatched to respond to a 36-year-old female with injuries after a fall. The dispatcher tells you the patient fell off the bed as she was getting into it. You are expecting this to be a pretty straightforward call, as falling from the edge of a bed, for an adult, is not likely to cause significant injuries. When you arrive, however, you are directed to your patient, Elizabeth, who is still on the ground and in obvious pain. Elizabeth tells you she has achondroplastic dwarfism and has broken several bones previously. A quick assessment reveals deformity, pain, and swelling of her left ankle from her fall, and also of her left arm and wrist where she tried to break her fall. You splint both injured areas and start an IV to administer pain medication. After asking Elizabeth the best way to help her move to the stretcher, she scoots onto a folded sheet placed on the floor, and she is carefully lifted to the stretcher.

Dwarfism is defined as having an adult height of 4′ 10″ or less. According to the Little People of America,[52] there are several terms that can be used appropriately to describe individuals with dwarfism including *dwarf, little person,* or *person of short stature.* The term "midget" is derogatory and never appropriate.

There are many genetic conditions that can lead to dwarfism, which is divided into two general categories, *proportionate dwarfism* and *disproportionate dwarfism.*[53] Proportionate dwarfism refers to a condition in which all body parts are small to the same degree, and the body is proportioned like one of average size/height. Disproportionate dwarfism refers to a condition in which some body parts are smaller than average, while others are average.

Little People of America notes that there are more than 200 types of dwarfism, but the most common types are the following: [54]

1. Achondroplasia (1 in 26,000 to 40,000 births and 70% of dwarfism cases)

2. Spondyloepiphyseal dysplasia congenita (1 in 95,000 births)

3. Diastrophic dysplasia (1 in 110,000 births)

Achondroplasia

Achondroplasia is the most common type of disproportionate dwarfism. The physical characteristics include short stature, average torso, shorter arms and legs, and a large head with a prominent forehead.[55] Although there are several potentially serious complications associated with achondroplasia, most people with this condition have a normal life expectancy.[56]

Pediatric complications associated with achondroplasia include the following:

- *Foramen magnum stenosis.* The *foramen magnum* is the hole at the bottom of the skull through which the spinal cord passes. In infants with achondroplasia, this opening can be too small, which can cause compression of the brain stem. The resulting brain stem compression can cause apnea, paralysis/paresis, and swallowing and feeding problems. The risk for sudden infant death in babies with achondroplasia is 2%–5%.[57] Foramen magnum stenosis can be treated by surgery if the symptoms are severe enough.

- *Spinal cord compression.* Compression of the spinal cord, especially at the junction of the brainstem and the cervical spine just below the foramen magnum, is common in infants in achondroplasia and can be responsible for paralysis, central and obstructive apnea, respiratory distress, and death.[58] Spinal cord compression in the thoracic or lumbar regions of the spine can cause paraplegia.[59]

- *Sleep disturbances and obstructive and central sleep apnea in children.* As many as 85% of children with achondroplasia can experience sleep apnea in some form, possibly due to airway *malacia*, or collapsible cartilage in the airway that can compromise its patency.[60] This can result in the need for medical interventions such as supplemental oxygen, CPAP, adenoidectomy, tonsillectomy, or tracheostomy.[61] In addition to the potentially life-threatening breathing issues associated with obstructive sleep apnea, children with achondroplasia and sleep disturbances also experienced daytime sleepiness, trouble with attention and concentration, behavior problems, and headaches.[62]

- *Hydrocephalus.* Hydrocephalus can occur throughout the lifespan, but the risk is greatest in the first two years of life.[63] (See the section on spina bifida for more information on hydrocephalus.)

- *Frequent ear infections.* Children with achondroplasia are considerably more likely to have abnormal middle ear function resulting in otitis media, or middle ear infections, as well as conductive hearing loss.[64]

- *Thoracolumbar kyphosis*. This is an outward curvature of the thoracic spine (hunchback) that can result in the need for surgical correction or braces.

As the individual with achondroplasia grows, there can be additional complications:

- *Spinal stenosis*. A narrowing, or *stenosis*, of the spine can compress the spinal cord and cause numbness and weakness.[65] This condition can result from thoracolumbar kyphosis.

- *Bowing of the legs*. This can lead to difficulty walking and an increased risk of falls, as well as chronic pain.[66]

- *Reflux*. Gastroesophageal reflux can cause pain and discomfort.[67]

- *Obesity*. Obesity affects about 50% of people with achondroplasia. In addition to the obvious risks of obesity, people with achondroplasia are at increased risk for bone and joint damage due to increased weight-bearing on fragile bones and joints. Obesity also increases the risk for cardiovascular problems, obstructive sleep apnea, and high cholesterol.[68]

- *Low bone density*. This is possibly due to changes in bone metabolism inherent to achondroplasia (see the section on spinal cord injuries for more information on the impact of low bone density).[69]

Surgical options for people with achondroplasia

- *Limb lengthening*. Some people with achondroplasia may elect to have surgery to lengthen their legs. One study reports the average increase in length is slightly more than 8 centimeters for the femur and slightly under 10 centimeters for the tibia.[70] Complications from the surgery that could contribute to the need for a postoperative EMS response include infection, fractures, and pain.

- *Cervical or thoracic spine fusion*. Instability or dislocation of the vertebrae can result in the need for surgical repair. Postoperatively, the patient may need to wear a halo device. The halo encircles the head and is secured by surgically implanted pins. The halo is stabilized to the body with a rigid vest or brace. The halo may be worn for several months as the bones heal after surgery. Wearing the halo can increase a child's risk of falling, resulting in injuries requiring an emergency transport. If the child has a car seat that is able to accommodate the halo device, be sure to transport using that car seat, if possible.

An emergency response can be complicated if the call is for a malfunctioning halo device (it breaks or becomes dislodged) or if the patient has experienced a significant mechanism of injury (e.g., ground level fall, motor vehicle accident) that can cause additional damage to the halo, the patient, or both (see fig. 5–2). In these cases, consider calling a pediatric base station or adult trauma center (depending on the age of the patient and circumstances of the event) for physician orders on what to do with a damaged halo device and plan for transport to a trauma center.

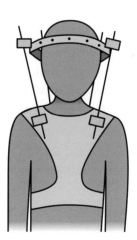

Fig. 5–2. A halo device

Spondyloepiphyseal dysplasia congenita

People with the bone growth disorder *spondyloepiphyseal dysplasia congenita* have a short trunk, neck, and limbs with average-sized hands and feet. Spine curvatures are common in childhood, and cervical vertebrae are unstable, leading to spinal cord damage. The chest is often barrel-shaped, leading to breathing difficulties. Other symptoms may include club foot, cleft palate, nearsightedness, and hearing loss.[71]

Diastrophic dysplasia

Diastrophic dysplasia is a type of dwarfism affects cartilage and bone development. People with diastrophic dysplasia have short stature as well as short arms and legs, early onset of osteoarthritis, progressively worsening scoliosis, clubfoot, finger deformities, cleft palate, and deformed ears.[72]

Implications for EMS

- Nighttime airway complications can be common in children with dwarfism. While there may not be much a prehospital provider can do other than general airway management and support, these events can be frightening for parents, and they may call 911. Be prepared to intervene and support as necessary.

- The patient's arm may not fully extend at the elbow, making IV insertion difficult.[73]

- Be prepared to assist patients with accessing the stretcher or ambulance. Ask them how they would like to be assisted. Do not pick them up without their permission. Whenever possible and medically appropriate, lower the stretcher as much as possible to allow for independent access.

- Provide additional padding and support for the patient on the stretcher to accommodate for limbs or joints that do not bend easily or typically.

- Assess the patient carefully as they are at greater risk for injury after a fall or other traumatic event.

- Patients with temporary surgical implants (e.g., pins from a halo device) are at greater risk for infection and sepsis.

- Skin breakdown can occur under the vest or brace supporting a halo device. This can cause pain and discomfort.

Ehlers-Danlos Syndrome

You are en route after being dispatched for a 22-year-old female with injuries after a fall. You arrive on scene at the local community college, and public safety directs you to the patient, Susan, sitting on the ground, surrounded by her friends. After you ask her friends to step back so she can have some privacy, Susan tells you she has vascular Ehlers-Danlos syndrome and she is unstable on her feet, falling often. Today she tripped going up the stairs and landed on her abdomen on one of the steps. She also landed on her wrist, dislocating it.

You quickly help Susan to the stretcher and into the ambulance to perform a thorough physical assessment. While your partner splints her wrist, you conduct a head-to-toe physical assessment. Palpation of her abdomen reveals that it is tender and slightly distended. Even though the fall appeared to be minor, you know that people with vascular Ehlers-Danlos syndrome are at increased risk for internal bleeding after a fall. Based on this knowledge, you prepare to transport Susan to a trauma center.

Ehlers-Danlos syndrome[74] is comprised of a collection of genetic connective tissue disorders, first described in 1901 and in the literature for decades.[75] Ehlers-Danlos syndrome primarily affects the skin and joints but can have other significant complications that may necessitate an EMS response. According to the National Institutes of Health, the prevalence of all types of Ehlers-Danlos syndrome as 1 in 5,000 people, with some of the variants being very rare, with only a few cases reported.[76] Although there are several subtypes of Ehlers-Danlos syndrome, the more common types are classic (11%), hypermobility (71%), and vascular (7%). Other subtypes make up the remaining 8%.[77]

Classic type

The characteristics of the classic variant of Ehlers-Danlos syndrome include joint hypermobility and fragile skin that stretches and is easily damaged and bruised, which may result in significant scarring. Other characteristics include slow wound healing, muscle cramps, and fatigue. Joint hypermobility causes joints that are easily dislocated and unstable. The extension and fragile nature of tissue throughout the body can lead to hernias and rectal prolapse.[78]

Gastrointestinal symptoms are common, with the most frequently occurring symptoms being nausea, vomiting, heartburn, constipation, and diarrhea.[79]

Pregnancy can cause challenges for women with the classic form of Ehlers-Danlos syndrome. Premature membrane rupture can occur, contributing to early delivery and a premature baby. Skin fragility can lead to skin tearing or a need for a larger episiotomy incision. Uterine prolapse can also occur. Babies who have Ehlers-Danlos syndrome while in utero have a higher incidence of breech presentation and dislocation of joints during delivery.

Vascular type

The vascular type has similar, yet more severe, issues with skin and joint fragility than the classic type. More concerning, however, are the vascular complications associated with tissue fragility. These vascular complications include arterial dissection, aneurysm, and/or rupture. Two-thirds of arterial ruptures occur in the thorax or abdomen, with the remaining one-third equally distributed between the head, neck, and extremities.[80]

Gastrointestinal perforation can occur in those with vascular Ehlers-Danlos syndrome. The majority of the ruptures occur in the colon, but ruptures can be experienced in the stomach and small intestine as well. Intestinal rupture can lead to sepsis. Less serious gastrointestinal symptoms include nausea, vomiting, heartburn, and constipation.[81]

People with vascular Ehlers-Danlos syndrome have also been found to be at risk for poor coagulation and may bleed excessively following injury, both internally and externally, and may require the use of thrombocytic and clot-formation substances.[82]

If your patient with Ehlers-Danlos syndrome shows signs or symptoms of hypovolemia or is otherwise hemodynamically unstable, consider internal bleeding secondary to arterial or peritoneal hemorrhage[83] and be prepared to treat external bleeding aggressively.[84]

Spontaneous and recurrent *pneumothorax* or *hemothorax* (collapsed lung due to air or blood between chest wall and lung, respectively) is possible and can result in difficulty breathing and bleeding from ruptured blood vessels within the lungs.[85]

Pregnancy for women with vascular Ehlers-Danlos syndrome can be dangerous and possibly fatal due to arterial dissection, uterine rupture, and surgical complications. One study reported on 35 women with a combined total of 76 deliveries.[86] Of those deliveries, approximately 48% were without complications. Of the 35 women, 5 died either during pregnancy, during labor/delivery, or in the immediate postpartum period, with 4 of those deaths due to aortic or other arterial rupture. Other nonfatal complications included arterial dissection, uterine rupture, preterm delivery, perineal lacerations, and hemorrhage requiring transfusion.

Vascular Ehlers-Danlos syndrome can be life-threatening. The average age of patients experiencing an arterial or gastrointestinal complication is 23 years, with 80% experiencing a life-threatening complication by age 40.[87] Being able to not only recognize Ehlers-Danlos complications in the prehospital setting but also to know how to treat them can help reduce mortality and morbidity for these patients.

Hypermobility type

The hypermobility variant of Ehlers-Danlos syndrome is the most frequent and the least severe.[88] It is also called *joint hypermobility syndrome*.[89] Common symptoms include unstable joints, easily damaged tissues, and chronic pain. Chronic fatigue and poor sleep are also common, thought to be associated with the chronic pain.[90]

Other characteristics of the hypermobility variant include cardiovascular manifestations (palpitations, dizziness, and syncope), gastrointestinal manifestations (reflux, general gastrointestinal discomfort, and irritable bowel syndrome), easy bruising and bleeding, painful menstrual cycles, stress urinary incontinence, fecal incontinence, and headaches.[91]

Psychiatric issues are also common, especially depression and anxiety related to living with chronic pain[92] and a reduced quality of life.[93] Murray et al.[94] reported 73% of patients with hypermobility-type Ehlers-Danlos syndrome experienced anxiety, and 69% experienced depression. More than three-quarters (82%) experienced chronic fatigue. Living with chronic pain, especially with a disorder that may be difficult to diagnose and differentiate from other chronic pain disorders, can have a significantly negative effect on one's quality of life.

Implications for EMS

- These patients will need to be moved carefully. Be sure to ask the most appropriate way to lift and move them in order to reduce the risk of joint dislocation.

- Skin tears can result in large wounds that need multiple layers of stitches and may bleed significantly, requiring direct pressure and hemostatic dressings.
- Be prepared to consider pain management for dislocated joints.
- Unexplained, new onset of pain requires immediate attention and assessment for arterial rupture.
- Consider internal bleeding for hemodynamically unstable patients with no known cause other than a diagnosis of Ehlers-Danlos syndrome.
- Consider sepsis due to bowel perforation for patients who meet physiological sepsis criteria (tachycardia, tachypnea, hypocapnia, fever) but do not have an obvious source of infection.
- Take all complaints of chest pain seriously, even in those patients not typically associated with cardiovascular disease (young and female), as it could indicate an arterial dissection.
- Abdominal pain may signal an intestinal rupture or perforation.
- Assess women in labor carefully and transport expeditiously.
- Minimize invasive procedures and antiplatelet drugs (such as aspirin) unless absolutely necessary to avoid EMS-induced injury or perforation.[95]

Osteogenesis Imperfecta

You are dispatched to an elementary school for traumatic injuries in a 10-year-old boy. School personnel direct you to the playground, where you find your patient, Scott, sitting by the climbing equipment, supporting his left arm. He is alert and oriented but in obvious pain. He tells you he has a diagnosis of osteogenesis imperfecta, type I (which the school nurse confirms and notes that Scott's parents have been notified) and tripped on the playground, landing on his left side. As you begin your assessment, you see his left forearm bent at a 45° angle. There is also swelling between the elbow and shoulder. You splint for stability and establish IV access in his right arm for pain management and transport him to the nearest pediatric facility for definitive care.

Osteogenesis imperfecta, also known as "brittle bone disease," is character-ized by bones that are very fragile and break easily, sometimes for no apparent reason. Osteogenesis imperfecta is an inherited disorder of connective tissue with abnormalities of the bone protein collagen.[96]

Osteogenesis imperfecta affects 1 per 20,000 live births,[97] with an estimated 25,000 to 50,000 people affected in the United States.[98] The Osteogenesis Imperfecta Foundation describes eight different types of osteogenesis imper-fecta with varying degrees of severity,[99] although new variants continue to be identified.[100] Table 5–2 describes the types of osteogenesis imperfecta and their relative severity.

Table 5–2. Types of osteogenesis imperfecta

Types of Osteogenesis Imperfecta	
Type	**Characteristics/Severity**
I	• Most common and least severe type.
	• More fractures occur before puberty.
	• Average stature.
	• Loose joints and muscle weakness.
	• Tendency to scoliosis (spine curvature).
	• Hearing loss can occur in young adulthood.
	• May have brittle teeth.
	• Blue, purple, or gray color to the *sclera* (whites of the eyes).
II	• Most severe form.
	• Fractures can occur before birth.
	• Death frequently occurs at birth or within a few weeks.
	• Lungs are not fully developed.
	• Significant bone deformities.
	• Blue, purple, or gray color to the sclera.
III	• Most severe type in children who survive the neonatal period.
	• Breathing and swallowing problems are common.
	• Fractures may be present before or at birth.
	• Adult stature is usually shorter than 3½ feet.
	• Rib and long bone fractures are common.
	• Spine and chest deformities are frequent.
	• Bone deformities may be severe and progressive.

Table 5–2. ...*continued*

III **cont'd**	• May have brittle teeth. • Hearing loss is common. • Blue, purple, or gray color to the sclera.
IV	• More severe than type I but less severe than type III. • Fractures may not occur until the child is walking. • Height is shorter than average. • Bone deformities may be mild to moderate. • Spine and chest deformities may be present. • May have brittle teeth. • May have hearing loss.
V	• Similar to type IV in frequency of fractures and the degree of bone deformity. • Large calluses, or areas of new bone growth, are seen at fracture and surgical sites. • Calluses may also appear spontaneously.
VI	• Very rare. • Similar in presentation to type V with moderate-to-severe deformities. • Bone differences are seen at the microscopic level.
VII	• Some cases are similar to type IV in appearance and symptoms. • Moderate to severe deformities. • Other cases are more like type II. • Stature is short. • Shorter than average humerus and femur. • Possible deformities in the hips.
VIII	• Resembles type II or type III in appearance and symptoms. • Severe growth deficiency is present. • Extreme undermineralization of the skeleton.

Sources: Justin E. Sam and Mala Dharmalingam, "Osteogenesis Imperfecta," *Indian Journal of Endocrinology and Metabolism*, 21, no. 6 (2017): 903, https://doi.org/10.4103/ijem. ijem_220_17; Fratzl-Zelman et al., "Classification of Osteogenesis Imperfecta," *Wiener Medizinische Wochenschrift* 165, no. 13–14 (2015): 264–270, https://doi.org/10.1007/s10354-015-0368-3; US Dept. of Health and Human Services, National Institutes of Health, "Osteogenesis Imperfecta Overview," Osteoporosis and Related Bone Diseases National Resource Center, May 2015, Publication No. 15–AR–8004, retrieved December 31, 2017, https://www.bones.nih.gov/sites/bones/files/overview_oi.pdf; and Osteogenesis Imperfecta Foundation, "Types of OI," 2015, retrieved December 31, 2017, http://www.oif.org/site/PageServer?pagename=AOI_Types.

Patients who have discoloration of the sclera may be predisposed to glaucoma and cataracts. Because osteogenesis is a disorder of collagen production, patients are also at risk for problems with cardiac and aortic valves.[101]

Treatments for osteogenesis imperfecta include medical and surgical management with the goals of reducing fractures and pain and increasing mobility and growth.[102] Medications aim to increase bone volume and density and reduce fractures.[103] Surgical interventions can include the insertion of rods in long bones to stabilize them and spinal fusions to address scoliosis and improve pulmonary function.[104] Patients may also have a halo device for cervical stability.[105]

Child abuse or osteogenesis imperfecta?

Because of the frequency of fractures and bruising associated with osteogenesis imperfecta, it can look like the injuries of child abuse. The role of EMS providers is not to investigate or make a determination if child abuse has taken place. If a child has fractures that seem inconsistent with events (e.g., a femur fracture after a ground level fall), it must be a consideration, especially as the incidence of fractures resulting from child abuse is considerably higher than of osteogenesis imperfecta.[106]

Physical and radiological findings that are more commonly seen in a non-accidental injury (abuse) include the following:[107]

- Bruises on the back, ears, and genitals
- Abdominal trauma (especially accompanied by fractures)
- Traumatic brain injury without skull fracture
- Symmetrical rib fractures
- Fractures toward the ends of long bones (*metaphyseal fractures*)
- Skull fractures

Long bone fractures typically associated with osteogenesis imperfecta are midshaft.[108]

EMS providers who suspect child abuse should report their concerns according to local protocols and document all observed injuries carefully in their patient care report, being cautious to report observations objectively and without judgment. The determination of child abuse may not be able to be confirmed without x-rays and a thorough medical evaluation[109] and is not something that can be easily determined in the prehospital setting.

Implications for EMS

- Parents may carry documentation of the diagnosis as the injuries associated with osteogenesis imperfecta can be mistaken for child abuse.
- Recognize that even very minor injuries or falls can cause fractures.
- Be prepared to address pain management.
- Be very cautious when lifting and moving patients to avoid exacerbating injuries or creating new ones.
- Scoliosis and chest deformities can reduce pulmonary function, leading to pulmonary disease and respiratory infections.[110]
- As many as 50% of adult patients may have hearing loss, so ensure that your patient has heard you, especially in a noisy environment.[111]
- Some children may have a cerebral shunt for hydrocephalus.[112] (See section on spina bifida for more discussion about shunts and shunt complications.)
- Surgical procedures carry the risk of postoperative infection. Consider sepsis in symptomatic postoperative patients.

Spina Bifida

You are dispatched to a local elementary school for an eight-year-old boy with altered mental status. You arrive on scene and meet your patient, Eli, in the nurse's office, alert but slow to respond. The nurse reports that he has spina bifida and a ventriculoperitoneal shunt. His symptoms started after arriving at school when his teacher noted he was not able to answer questions he typically could and seemed sleepy. When you ask Eli if he has any pain, he responds, "My head hurts," and promptly vomits on your shoes. You immediately suspect a shunt malfunction and prepare to transport emergently to a pediatric facility.

Spina bifida (literally "split spine") is a birth defect that occurs during the prenatal period, and it is present in approximately 1 to 2 cases per 1,000 people in the United States each year.[113] About 1,500 babies are born each year in the United States with the most serious form of spina bifida.[114] During early fetal development, the *neural tube*, which is an embryonic structure that becomes the central nervous system (brain and spinal cord), does not close properly. This can cause the *meninges* (the membrane covering the brain and spinal cord) and spinal cord to form outside of the baby's body cavity. Depending on the type of spina bifida and its severity, a variety of severe physical issues may result. The most common location for spina bifida is the lumbosacral region, followed by the thoracic region, and in rare cases, the cervical region.[115]

Risk factors for spina bifida

While most cases of spina bifida have no clear cause, some things have been shown to be possible risk factors, including family history, maternal diabetes, maternal obesity, maternal hyperthermia (from fever, saunas, and tanning beds), and insufficient folic acid (vitamin B-9).[116]

Types of Spina Bifida

Spina bifida occulta

In *spina bifida occulta*, there are no obvious outward signs of improper spine or spinal cord development, but a gap in the spine may be seen on x-ray. Spina bifida occulta typically does not cause any pain or disability (fig. 5–3).

Meningocele

Meningocele is a less severe form of spina bifida, but it is also less common, occurring in 1 in 5,000 births. In this type of spina bifida, the meninges, along with some cerebral spinal fluid, protrude from an opening in the back. The spinal cord remains inside the body. This condition is typically easily repaired in infancy with surgery, and long-lasting problems with pain and disability are uncommon.

Myelomeningocele

This form of spina bifida is more common, occurring in 1 in 800 births. In *myelomeningocele*, part of the spinal cord is outside of the body inside the protruding meninges. While myelomeningocele can be surgically corrected, the exposed spinal cord will be injured by the damaged vertebrae and irritation from amniotic fluid during pregnancy and before birth,[117] resulting in paralysis or paresis below the exposed area.

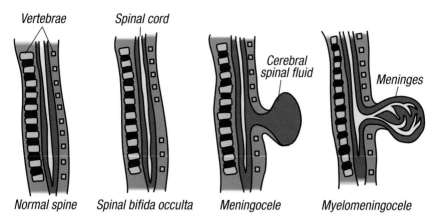

Fig. 5–3. Types of spina bifida

Special Concerns with Myelomeningocele Spina Bifida

The severity of spina bifida is dependent on the location of the opening in the spine and the subsequent spinal cord/nerve damage.

Paralysis

Paralysis is a frequent complication in people with spina bifida. The location and severity of the paralysis is directly related to the location of the lesion and exposure of the spinal cord. People with paralysis are at an increased risk of injury from falls and other accidents, especially when coupled with the decrease in bone density that is also common (see below). Another complication of paralysis is diminished or absent pain response. An individual may be injured and not recognize the injury, which can lead to further complications.

Chiari malformation

A *Chiari malformation* occurs when there is "herniation of the [cerebellar] tonsils and the contents of the posterior fossa into the foramen magnum."[118] This means that part of the *cerebellum* (the area of the brain that controls balance) and some of the brain stem protrude through the base of the skull and are compressed.[119] Four types of Chiari malformations occur with various levels of severity, with the Chiari II malformation being most closely associated with spina bifida.

A *Chiari II malformation* (also called an *Arnold-Chiari malformation*) occurs in 95% of people with spina bifida and is associated with a reduced life expectancy.[120] When symptomatic, it is the most common cause of death in children with spina bifida under the age of two years. A Chiari II malformation causes symptoms in up to one-third of those individuals, most commonly headaches, poor oral feeding, abnormal respiratory function/apnea, sleep apnea, vocal fold paralysis, abnormal eye movements, and weakness.[121] The feeding difficulties associated with a Chiari II malformation can result in failure to thrive and pulmonary aspiration. Symptomatic Chiari II malformations are treated surgically.[122]

Hydrocephalus

A common co-occurring condition associated with spina bifida is *hydrocephalus*, or literally "water on the head." As many as 70% to 90% of individuals with myelomeningocele spina bifida have hydrocephalus.[123] Cerebrospinal fluid normally circulates throughout the central nervous system to protect and cushion the brain and spinal cord, provide nutrients, and remove waste. Spina bifida can prevent the cerebrospinal fluid from draining or circulating properly. The fluid accumulates around the brain, causing increased pressure on the brain and possibly damage. In order to prevent this pressure-caused damage, a small, flexible tube called a shunt can be inserted into the ventricles or other spaces in the brain to drain the fluid into the abdomen (a *ventriculoperitoneal shunt*) or into the heart atria (a *ventriculoatrial shunt*)[124] to prevent buildup and subsequent complications. Authors of a recent study found a shunt placement prevalence of 56%.[125] Complications can occur postoperatively or at any time the shunt is in place.

Shunt complications

- *Postoperative infection.* As with any surgical procedure, a postoperative infection is a possible complication, typically happening within the first several weeks following the procedure. Signs and symptoms of a postoperative infection include fever, pain, and redness, swelling, or drainage from the incision.

- *Shunt dysfunction.* Shunts can break or become dislodged or blocked. A nonfunctioning shunt can be a medical emergency. Signs of a problem with a shunt include headache, vomiting/nausea, seizures (new or worsening), changes in speech, balance, or coordination, irritability, vision problems, sleepiness, or unusual behavior.[126]

- *Other complications.* While the insertion site for a shunt is in the ventricles of the brain, the distal end can be in the abdomen. The foreign body in the abdomen can cause pain and discomfort, bowel perforation or hernia, or *pseudocysts* (a collection of cerebrospinal fluid in the abdomen near the shunt potentially leading to pain, distension, or infection).[127]

Latex allergy

People with spina bifida are at increased risk for developing a latex allergy, potentially resulting in anaphylaxis. This is possibly due to a predisposition to the allergy coupled with early and repeated exposure to latex during surgeries and other medical procedures, along with the use of urinary catheters, gloves, and the like.[128] Those individuals who have a ventricular shunt are at even higher risk, even though the shunt itself is nonlatex,[129] because they have an increased risk of latex exposure due to frequent surgical procedures related to the shunt. One study, however, reported that the likelihood of developing a latex allergy "appears primarily related to the disease of spina bifida itself and only secondarily to the number of exposures to latex products," indicating that merely having spina bifida increases the risk for latex allergy, regardless of repeated latex exposure.[130]

Fewer individuals are developing a latex allergy now that the use of latex in the medical setting has decreased, however, and fewer children are becoming sensitized.[131] The prevalence of latex allergy varies by study but is reported to be as high as 55% for individuals with spina bifida (see table 5–3).[132] The prevalence of latex allergy in the general population is estimated at about 4%.[133]

While prehospital settings now generally use latex-free materials, and people with a latex allergy understand the need to avoid known sources of latex, it can still be found in hidden and unexpected places. People with latex allergies can have a reaction if they are touched by someone or something that has been in contact with latex without having direct contact themselves. For example, indirect reactions can be caused if the powder residue remains on someone's hands after they wear latex gloves and then touch someone else. It may be caused by a food service worker wearing latex gloves while preparing food that is then consumed by a person with a latex allergy. People can also be impacted by airborne latex particles. If a balloon pops, the latex powder inside the balloon will be released into the air.

Table 5–3. Latex allergy rate reports for people with spina bifida

Latex Allergy Rate Reports for People with Spina Bifida	
Nieto et al., 2000	44%
Michael et al., 1996	49%
Ausili et al., 2007	37%
Blumchen et al., 2010	55%

Sources: Blumchen et al., "Effects of Latex Avoidance on Latex Sensitization, Atopy and Allergic Diseases in Patients with Spina Bifida"; Ausili et al., "Prevalence of Latex Allergy in Spina Bifida: Genetic and Environmental Factors"; A. Nieto et al., "The Search of Latex Sensitization in Spina Bifida: Diagnostic Approach"; and Michael et al., "Risk Factors for Latex Allergy in Patients with Spina Bifida."

The Spina Bifida Association[134] provides helpful information about unfamiliar or hidden sources of latex. Some things that may contain latex (and may not be labeled as such) include chewing gum, playground and other sports balls, clothing elastic, shoes, nonslip handles on tools, pool/beach toys including swim goggles, toys (especially toy car wheels), and removable covers on the bottom of crutches or chair/table legs.

While most items on ambulances are latex free, such as gloves and IV supplies, there can still be sources of unexpected latex. This hidden latex may be found in your stethoscope tubing, adhesive bandages, the plunger tips of disposable syringes, or IV tourniquets. If you are unsure if a product contains latex, check the packaging, which should have a symbol or text indicating if the product is latex free (fig. 5–4).

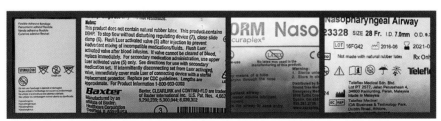

Fig. 5–4. Check labels for latex content because some people are allergic to latex.

Foods such as avocados, bananas, kiwis, potatoes, tomatoes, and chestnuts contain some of the same components as latex. They may cause an allergic reaction in as many as 50% of people who are also allergic to latex, with avocados and bananas being the most likely foods to cause anaphylaxis.[135]

If you are assessing and treating a patient with spina bifida, assume they have a latex allergy until told otherwise and avoid any patient contact with latex. Be sure to consider an inadvertent exposure to latex when your patient with spina bifida is showing signs/symptoms of an allergic reaction and possible anaphylaxis and be prepared to intervene accordingly.

Bladder problems

As a consequence of the spinal cord injury inherent in spina bifida, bladder dysfunction is common, resulting in urinary retention, incontinence, or *reflux* (urine backing up through the ureters into the kidneys), which can increase the risk of recurrent urinary tract infections.[136]

Regular/routine catheterization can also increase the risk of urinary tract infections. Urinary tract infections are one of the most common causes for hospital admission for people with spina bifida.[137] People with paralysis, paresis, or decreased sensation may be unaware of the developing urinary tract infection symptoms of pain, urgency, and frequency. These infections, if unnoticed and untreated, can lead to sepsis, which can be fatal. EMS providers will want to be especially cognizant of this possibility when assessing and treating patients with spina bifida who are showing signs and symptoms of a urinary tract infection or sepsis.

Skin breakdown

Skin breakdown and open wounds are frequent with spina bifida, occurring in as many as 85% to 95% of children with myelomeningocele.[138] Patients who use wheelchairs for mobility are at a higher risk for skin breakdown, and people with their spinal opening at the thoracic level have a higher incidence of open wounds than patients with lumbar or sacral involvement. Wounds are commonly found on the feet and ankles, followed by the buttocks and trunk.

Wounds occur for a variety of reasons. People who are able to walk may have reduced sensation in their feet and legs and thus may not be able to protect themselves as easily from injury. Diminished sensation can contribute to exposure contact injuries, which could include inadvertent immersion in scalding bath water or walking barefoot on surfaces that are too hot or too cold due to inability to accurately judge the temperature.[139] Pressure ulcers from immobilization in wheelchairs or beds are also common. Ulcers can be caused by any part of a wheelchair or bed that causes unusual pressure on the skin. Porter and Kelly report on one patient with spina bifida who had a pressure ulcer on the anterior surface of his torso caused by leaning against the tray of his wheelchair.[140]

Because people with spina bifida have reduced sensation, it is imperative that EMS providers use caution when lifting, moving, and positioning these patients on the stretcher. Be careful to avoid aggravating existing skin injuries and avoid contributing to new injury by rubbing, pinching, or otherwise irritating the skin, especially as the patient may not be aware of the irritation.

Low bone density

People with spina bifida have significantly lower bone mineral content and bone mineral density when compared to the general population. This subsequently causes an increased risk for osteoporosis and fractures.[141] Due to decreased sensation in the extremities, a fracture may go unnoticed initially, or it may not be the primary complaint. EMS providers need to be aware of this increased risk of fractures when assessing and treating patients with spina bifida who may have injuries.

Low impact mechanisms may cause injuries in patients with spina bifida that might not cause injuries in the general population, so when assessing, be cautious not to make assumptions about potential injury without doing a complete assessment. Also be aware that a typical pain assessment may not be possible, so look for other clinical signs of injury and err on the side of caution when deciding about stabilization and splinting an extremity. While one purpose of splinting is to reduce pain, splinting is also done to reduce the chance of exacerbating the current injury and causing more damage to the limb. Even if the patient is not complaining of pain, it may be necessary to splint a limb.

Risky behaviors

Soe et al. interviewed 130 young adults ages 16–31 years with spina bifida about their behaviors that could have a potential negative impact on their overall health and well-being.[142] These behaviors included poor eating habits, limited physical activity, and substance abuse (alcohol, cigarettes, illegal drugs). While many young adults without significant health concerns engage in these behaviors, the results from this study reveal that the individuals with spina bifida who participated in the study exhibited significantly higher rates of poor diet (75% versus 12% in the general population) and limited physical activity (74% versus 22% of the general population). Alcohol, cigarettes, and illegal drug use, however, were lower among the study participants with spina bifida when compared to the general population.

Bowel problems

Most people with spina bifida have difficulty with bowel function due to disruption in the nerves that innervate the rectum and anus.[143] As a result, both bowel incontinence and constipation are common.

Depression

In one study, almost half of the participants (48%) aged 16–31 years reported mild to significant depression, compared to 10% for the general population.[144] Major depressive symptoms were also associated with alcohol abuse. (See chapter 6, "Mental Health Disorders," for information on this population.)

Intellectual/learning disabilities

The rate of intellectual disability is higher in people with spina bifida, with one study reporting a prevalence of 19%[145] compared to the general population with a prevalence of 1% to 3%. The presence of hydrocephalus or a shunt is correlated with increased cognitive disabilities.[146] (See chapter 3 for information about intellectual disabilities.)

Obesity

People with spina bifida are at higher risk for obesity (estimated at 35% to 50%), not only due to limitations in mobility, including walking, that result in reduced activity levels, but also due to possible endocrine issues from hydrocephalus.[147] Obesity can lead to increased immobility and type II diabetes, as well as have detrimental effects on self-image and overall health.

Implications for EMS

- Patients who are injured may not be able to give you an accurate pain description due to paralysis or paresis. Be sure to conduct a thorough trauma assessment to uncover injuries they may not feel.

- Due to the increased risk for osteoporosis, be sure to consider fractures, even with low mechanism falls or mild injuries.

- There is an increased risk for sepsis due to the higher prevalence of urinary tract infections and pressure ulcers.

- Consider the potential for shunt malfunction if there is a sudden onset of headache, vomiting/nausea, seizures, changes in speech, balance, or coordination, irritability, vision problems, sleepiness, or unusual behavior.
- Don't forget to take mobility devices (crutches, walker, transport wheelchair) with you in the ambulance, if possible.

Spinal Cord Injuries: Paraplegia and Quadriplegia

You are dispatched for a 54-year-old male with an altered mental status and no other information. Upon your arrival, you locate your patient, James, lying on the ground near a swimming pool. He is conscious but initially slow to respond. You see a motorized wheelchair near the pool. James is with family members, and you notice he has nitroglycerin paste on his chest. As you ask questions, you learn that he has incomplete tetraplegia at the C5 level. He is able to ambulate a little with assistance but has diminished sensation to pain and temperature below the level of his injury. The water in the pool was colder than expected, and it caused autonomic dysreflexia, with a severe headache and a dangerously high rise in blood pressure. His son reported a manual blood pressure of 273/145 shortly after James got out of the pool, but it was coming down as he warmed up and with the application of the nitro paste.

After completion of the assessment, including a 12-lead EKG and vital signs, James agrees to be transported to the ED for further evaluation. At your prompting, he tells you the best way to help him move onto your stretcher. James is positioned sitting up and with pillows and blankets protecting him from further pinching, pressure, or other potentially irritating stimulus to prevent another blood pressure spike. You leave the nitro paste in place, monitoring his vitals while en route to watch for hypotension (not forgetting to take his transport wheelchair with you).

This section primarily considers spinal cord damage secondary to traumatic injury to the cord itself. Information on other causes of paralysis is available in the sections on spina bifida, cerebral palsy, and TBI.

The spinal cord can be damaged in a variety of ways, such as from a traumatic injury, stroke, tumors, spina bifida, or cerebral palsy, and may result in paraplegia or quadriplegia (also called *tetraplegia*). The prevalence of paralysis in the United States from any cause is estimated at 5.4 million people, with 72% younger than 65 years of age. Stroke is the leading cause of paralysis (almost 34% of those with paralysis), followed by spinal cord injury (27%).[148] There are approximately 276,000 people in the United States with a spinal cord injury, with more than 12,000 new cases each year.[149]

According to an article by Lawrence Chin, almost one-fourth of the patients who have a spinal cord injury do not survive past the event or the initial hospitalization.[150] The life expectancy for a patient with a spinal cord injury is below that of the general population. The leading causes of death are pneumonia, pulmonary embolism, and sepsis, with heart disease, trauma, suicide, and alcohol-related deaths as other major causes.

Types of injuries

The spinal column that protects the spinal cord is divided into four sections: cervical, thoracic, lumbar, and sacral/coccygeal (fig. 5–5). There are a total of 33 vertebrae, comprised of 7 cervical vertebrae, 12 thoracic, 5 lumbar, 5 sacral, and 4 (fused) coccygeal.[151] The severity of injury and degree of paralysis depend on the location of the injury, with higher level injuries typically being more severe. Quadriplegia occurs when the injury is above the first thoracic vertebra (T1), involving the cervical vertebrae (C1–C8). People with quadriplegia are unable to move their arms and legs (anything below the site of the injury). Injuries at the C1–C4 level are often fatal, and survivors of these high-level injuries will be unable to breathe on their own and may not be able to speak. People with injuries to the lower cervical spine (C5–C8) will still have paralysis below the site of injury resulting in quadriplegia but should be able to breath on their own and speak.

Paraplegia occurs when the injury involves the thoracic or lumbar vertebrae (T1–L5). People with paraplegia can use their arms and hands but may have leg paralysis or *paresis* (weakness). Injuries to the sacral region (S1–S5) typically do not result in paralysis or paresis but can cause problems with bladder or bowel functioning and with sexual functioning.

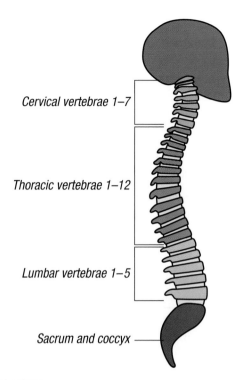

Fig. 5–5. Spinal column

Complete versus incomplete injuries

Spinal cord injury is also defined by the American Spinal Injury Association (ASIA) Impairment Scale.[152] ASIA describes five categories, differentiating between complete and incomplete injuries:

A = **Complete.** No sensory or motor function is preserved in sacral segments S4–S5.

B = **Sensory incomplete.** Sensory, but not motor, function is preserved below the neurologic level of injury and extends through sacral segments S4–S5.

C = **Motor incomplete.** Motor function is preserved below the neurologic level of injury, and most key muscles below the neurologic level of injury have a muscle grade of *less than 3* (table 5–4).

D = **Motor incomplete.** Motor function is preserved below the neurologic level of injury, and most key muscles below the neurologic level of injury have a muscle grade that is *greater than or equal to 3*.

E = **Normal.** Sensory and motor functions are normal.

Table 5–4. Muscle function grading

Muscle Function Grading	
0	Total paralysis
1	Palpable or visible contraction
2	Active movement, full range of motion with gravity eliminated
3	Active movement, full range of motion against gravity
4	Active movement, full range of motion against gravity and moderate resistance in a muscle specific position
5	Normal, active movement, full range of motion against gravity and full resistance in a functional muscle position expected from an otherwise unimpaired person

Source: American Spinal Injury Association and the International Spinal Cord Society, "Muscle Function Grading," *International Standards for Neurological Classification of Spinal Cord Injury* (ASIA and ISCS, 2015), http://asia-spinalinjury.org/wp-content/uploads/2016/02/International_Stds_Diagram_Worksheet.pdf.

Simply speaking, complete spinal cord injuries result in the absence of any motor or sensory functioning below the injury. Incomplete injuries can result in the preservation of sensory (including pain and temperature) and motor function to varying degrees below the level of the injury.

Specific types of incomplete spinal cord injuries include anterior cord syndrome, Brown-Séquard syndrome, and central cord syndrome.[153]

- *Anterior cord syndrome.* This is an injury to the anterior part of the spinal cord, which results in loss of motor function and temperature and pain sensation below the injury but preservation of the sensations of touch, vibration, and proprioception (or the sense of one's body positioning).

- *Brown-Séquard syndrome.* This is an injury to half of the spinal cord, which results in paralysis and loss of touch, vibration, and proprioception sensation on the same side as the injury, and loss of pain and temperature sensation on the opposite side.

- *Central cord syndrome.* This injury involves the cervical spine and is manifested by motor paralysis or weakness and loss of sensation (pain, temperature, vibration, touch, or proprioception) in the arms and hands. The lower extremities are affected to a lesser degree than the upper extremities.

Spinal cord injury complications

In addition to limb paralysis, secondary effects of spinal cord injury above T6 can be significant, resulting in cardiac, respiratory, urinary, gastrointestinal, and thermoregulatory complications that can result in emergency transport to the emergency department.[154]

Respiratory complications

High cervical injuries can impact functioning of the diaphragm, requiring mechanical ventilation or diaphragmatic pacing. Operational failure of either can result in the need for emergency breathing support. Additionally, because of thoracic paralysis, patients have generally ineffective respiration that results in atelectasis and pneumonia.[155] EMS providers should be cognizant of respiratory symptoms and treat according to their protocols.

Blood pressure abnormalities (autonomic dysreflexia)

As many as 90% of patients with a spinal cord injury at or above the T6 level can experience *autonomic dysreflexia (AD)*,[156] which is acute, uncontrolled hypertension that is potentially life-threatening and requires immediate treatment. It is triggered by a strong and/or unpleasant stimulus and can cause a rapid and dangerous rise in blood pressure at least 15 to 20 mmHg systolic above the patient's baseline, but it has been recorded as high as 250 to 300 mmHg.[157] It can also be associated with bradycardia. Higher levels of injury and increased severity of cord injury are associated with greater prevalence of autonomic dysreflexia.[158] Note that people with spinal cord injuries typically have low blood pressures, so a systolic pressure of 130 to 135 can be indicative of AD.

Autonomic dysreflexia can be triggered by anything below the level of the spinal cord injury that is painful, traumatic, unpleasant, and/or strong (like contact with a hard object). It is most commonly triggered, however, by urinary bladder irritation or distention (75%–85%) or bowel distention (13%–19%). Warning signs and symptoms of AD can range from mild to severe and include headache, nausea, confusion, anxiety, blurred vision, and facial flushing, with *diaphoresis* (excessive sweating) above the site of the injury and pale, cool skin and *piloerection* (goosebumps) below the level of injury. This is a potentially life-threatening condition since the risks for cerebral hemorrhage, cardiac dysrhythmias, retinal detachment, and seizures are high.[159]

Prevention of autonomic dysreflexia starts with avoidance of potential triggers through careful health management. Steps could include a daily bowel program to avoid constipation, regularly scheduled catheterization or Foley checks to avoid a full bladder, and also being aware of sources of injury and pain.

If you suspect a person has AD, check when they were last catheterized or if their Foley catheter is kinked or otherwise blocked. Ask when their last bowel program was done and if it emptied the colon. Once bladder and bowel causes have been ruled out, helping the person to sit upright may result in a reduction in blood pressure due to orthostatic changes. It is also important to loosen tight clothing or braces and look for unexpected stimuli.

Autonomic dysreflexia in a patient with no apparent trigger can be a clue for EMS providers to consider an undetected injury that has gone untreated. Kriz, Andel, and Hakova report on a patient who developed autonomic dysreflexia several days after what was described as a mild fall from his wheelchair with no obvious signs of injury.[160] After a careful review of his history of the previous several days, the fall was noted, and a CT scan revealed multiple pelvic fractures. The fractures were treated and the autonomic dysreflexia resolved. Although the primary concern for the prehospital provider would be addressing the hypertension, taking a thorough history can help the health care providers in the emergency department consider and treat all issues, including the presenting symptoms as well as the underlying cause.

Prehospital medical treatment includes frequent blood pressure monitoring and rapid onset/short duration antihypertensive medications such as nitrates, nifedipine, and captopril.[161] Consult your jurisdiction's protocols and obtain medical consultation before attempting to reduce blood pressure in the prehospital setting.

EMS providers should be aware of this potentially life-threatening complication to a medical or traumatic event in patients with spinal cord injuries and quadriplegia. While they may not be able to prevent autonomic dysreflexia, due to the common causes of bladder and colon irritation, they can be cautious not to trigger it through inadvertently causing irritation below the injury site through careful movement, positioning, and avoiding painful interventions, such as IV insertion, whenever possible. EMS providers should also be prepared to conduct a thorough medical and/or trauma assessment, take a full and complete history, and be prepared to refer and transport their patients with a history of spinal cord injuries and potential complications to a specialty center.

Deep vein thrombosis

A *deep vein thrombosis* (*DVT*), or blood clot, is a common complication of spinal cord injuries due to the immobility that is inherent with paralysis. People with spinal cord injuries are at greater risk for developing a DVT due to reduced vascular contraction and reduced venous blood return secondary to paralysis.[162] DVTs are more commonly found in the lower extremities and pelvis (85%); however, they can also occur in the upper extremities.[163]

While DVTs have been found in patients while they were still hospitalized for their initial injury, DVTs can occur at any time and can lead to a potentially fatal pulmonary embolism. EMS providers should consider the possibility of a DVT if their patient presents with redness or swelling in an extremity, as well as ask about possible DVT history in a patient who is presenting with signs and symptoms of a pulmonary embolism (sudden onset of shortness of breath, sudden chest pain, low SpO_2, tachycardia, tachypnea, and bloody/pink, frothy sputum).

Urologic and bowel problems

People with spinal cord injuries resulting in paralysis can have significant urologic issues such as problems with urine retention, incontinence, and elevated bladder pressure. Intermittent catheterization will be necessary, although an indwelling Foley catheter or suprapubic tube may also be in place. Urinary tract infections are extremely common, described by McGuire as "universal" in any patient who catheterizes regularly, regardless of type of catheter.[164] Remember that urinary retention or catheter problems can cause autonomic dysreflexia and a dangerous spike in blood pressure.[165] EMS providers should be aware of signs of urinary tract infection or other complications that may lead to autonomic dysreflexia or sepsis.

Risk of fractures

People with a spinal cord injury are at greater risk for developing osteoporosis and subsequently have an increased risk of fracture. As many as 80% of people with a spinal cord injury develop osteoporosis or its precursor, osteopenia. *Osteoporosis* occurs when bones lose density and become weak due to an imbalance between the creation of new bone cells and the absorption of old cells.[166]

Bone density below the level of the injury can start to diminish as early as six weeks after the injury and can continue to decrease for about two years. This decrease in bone density can contribute to fractures.

Several factors can contribute to osteoporosis in this population.[167] The most common is the lack of weight bearing on the bones, which is needed for cell generation. Interestingly, the spine typically maintains adequate bone density because of the weight bearing that occurs from sitting in a wheelchair. The legs, however, are at great risk due to disuse, losing as much as 40% of their density. Other issues that can contribute to osteoporosis after a spinal cord injury are poor circulation to the limbs, changes in hormone secretion, metabolic disturbances, and nervous system dysregulation, all related and secondary to the injury.

EMS providers need to be aware of this considerable increase in the risk of fractures. Be cautious when assessing patients for injury after an event that has the potential to cause a fracture, even if it does not appear to be significant enough to cause a fracture in a person without a spinal cord injury, such as a fall from a wheelchair or a low-speed, low-impact motor vehicle accident. EMS providers will typically consider mechanism of injury, patient reports of pain, or obvious injury/deformity to the body when considering severity of injury and possible fracture. When a patient has a spinal cord injury, however, do not assume there is no fracture just because there is minor mechanism, a lack of pain, or no obvious injury. Err on the side of caution and remember that the patient is at greater risk for fracture and should be treated and transported appropriately.

EMS providers must also be cautious when moving patients with spinal cord injuries, as they cannot tell you if something hurts, if their limbs are caught in the bed or wheelchair, or if they are not positioned comfortably. It is important not to inadvertently cause or exacerbate an injury.

Implications for EMS

- If possible, bring the patient's wheelchair in the ambulance. If their regular chair is too large or heavy, ask about a collapsible transport chair. Also be prepared to transport (or arrange to transport) a service animal.

- Ask the patient (or their family if they are unable to speak) about the best way to lift and move them. Do not pick them up without asking permission. In addition to being disrespectful, you can also cause additional damage. Remember that they may have a colostomy, urostomy, suprapubic catheter, or Foley catheter, along with a collection bag. Be cautious not to dislodge any of these items. Some people with spinal cord injuries cannot lie flat, so be sure to ask about their preferred position of comfort.

- Do not lift the person *in* the wheelchair, as the wheelchairs are typically not designed to be lifted.

- Pad all areas carefully to reduce the risk of pressure ulcers from the stretcher and the risk of autonomic dysreflexia from pinching or other discomfort. Pillows or padding under the arms and legs and behind the neck can aid in comfort.

- Keep patients experiencing autonomic dysreflexia sitting upright.

- Watch for limbs dangling off the stretcher or positioned awkwardly.

- Ask about bladder and bowel care, especially if conducting a long transport between facilities or between home and hospital. Be prepared to address leakage.

- Ask about their type of injury and if they have a complete or incomplete injury. Do not assume that they have no motor or sensory functioning, as that can vary widely.

- Be sure to get a complete list of medications, both prescribed and over the counter (including supplements), and don't forget to ask about alcohol and drug use. Don't assume because they are paralyzed that there can be no drug or alcohol use.

- Ask what their baseline blood pressure is, as it often tends to be low in people with spinal cord injuries. A blood pressure that is typically not concerning for most people (systolic in the 130s) can indicate autonomic dysreflexia in a person with a spinal cord injury.

- Some people who use wheelchairs prefer to be on the same level as the people they are talking to, so you might consider crouching down to talk with them face to face. Others, however, don't find it necessary, and it might even make them uncomfortable. Follow their cues and watch what people who are familiar with the patient do when making the decision whether to stand or crouch while speaking with your patient.[168] If possible, you could sit on a chair, which can be more natural.

Notes

1. John K. Spender, "On Some of the Rarer Complications of Rheumatoid Arthritis," *The British Medical Journal* 1, no. 1,635 (1892): 905–907.

2. J. A. Rindfleisch and D. Muller, "Diagnosis and Management of Rheumatoid Arthritis," *American Family Physician* 72, no. 6 (2005): 1,037–1,047, http://www.aafp.org/afp.

3. Rindfleisch and Muller, "Diagnosis and Management of Rheumatoid Arthritis"; J. Clements, "Treatment of Rheumatoid Arthritis: A Review of Recommendations and Emerging Therapy," *Formulary* 46 (2011): 532–545; and Matthias Schneider and Klaus Krüger, "Rheumatoid Arthritis—Early Diagnosis and Disease Management," *Deutsches Ärzteblatt International* 110, no. 27–28 (2013): 477–484.

4. William C. Shiel, Jr., "Rheumatoid Arthritis Treatment, RA Symptoms, Diagnosis, and Causes," November 16, 2017, retrieved December 30, 2017, https://www.medicinenet.com/rheumatoid_arthritis/article.htm.

5. S. Naz et al., "Juvenile Rheumatoid Arthritis," *Journal of the College of Physicians and Surgeons Pakistan* 23, no. 6 (2013): 409–412.

6. Shiel, Jr., "Rheumatoid Arthritis Treatment, RA Symptoms, Diagnosis, and Causes"; and Rindfleisch and Muller, "Diagnosis and Management of Rheumatoid Arthritis."

7. Shiel, Jr., "Rheumatoid Arthritis Treatment, RA Symptoms, Diagnosis, and Causes"; and Rindfleisch and Muller, "Diagnosis and Management of Rheumatoid Arthritis."

8. Shiel, Jr., "Rheumatoid Arthritis Treatment, RA Symptoms, Diagnosis, and Causes."

9. Clements, "Treatment of Rheumatoid Arthritis."

10. Rindfleisch and Muller, "Diagnosis and Management of RA."

11. Shiel, Jr., "Rheumatoid Arthritis Treatment, RA Symptoms, Diagnosis, and Causes"; Jose U. Scher et al., "Periodontal Disease and the Oral Microbiota in New-Onset Rheumatoid Arthritis," *Arthritis & Rheumatism* 64, no. 10 (2012): 3,083–3,094, https://doi.org/10.1002/art.34539; and Clements, "Treatment of Rheumatoid Arthritis."

12. Rindfleisch and Muller, "Diagnosis and Management of Rheumatoid Arthritis"; Clements, "Treatment of Rheumatoid Arthritis"; and Schneider and Krüger, "Rheumatoid Arthritis—Early Diagnosis and Disease Management."

13. US Department of Health and Human Services, Centers for Disease Control and Prevention, "Arthritis: Osteoarthritis," April 3, 2018, retrieved June 11, 2018, https://www.cdc.gov/arthritis/basics/osteoarthritis.htm.

14. Shiel, Jr., "Rheumatoid Arthritis Treatment, RA Symptoms, Diagnosis, and Causes"; William C. Shiel, Jr., "Osteoarthritis Treatment, Symptoms, Signs, & Causes," December 13, 2017, retrieved December 30, 2017, https://www.medicinenet.com/osteoarthritis/article.htm; and US Department of Health and Human Services, National Institutes of Health, National Institute of Arthritis and Musculoskeletal and Skin Diseases, "Osteoarthritis," May 20, 2016, retrieved June 11, 2018, https://www.niams.nih.gov/health-topics/osteoarthritis/advanced.

15. Shiel, Jr., "Rheumatoid Arthritis Treatment, RA Symptoms, Diagnosis, and Causes"; and Shiel, Jr., "Osteoarthritis Treatment, Symptoms, Signs, & Causes."

16. Shiel, Jr., "Rheumatoid Arthritis Treatment, RA Symptoms, Diagnosis, and Causes"; Shiel, Jr., "Osteoarthritis Treatment, Symptoms, Signs, & Causes"; Carlos J. Lozada, "Osteoarthritis Treatment and Management," Medscape.com, August 3, 2019, retrieved September 17, 2019, https://emedicine.medscape.com/article/330487-treatment; and US Dept. of HHS, NIH, NIAMS, "Osteoarthritis."

17. Shiel, Jr., "Osteoarthritis Treatment, Symptoms, Signs, & Causes"; and US Dept. of HHS, NIH, NIAMS, "Osteoarthritis."

18. Shiel Jr., "Osteoarthritis Treatment, Symptoms, Signs, & Causes"; and B. J. Messinger-Rapport and H. L. Thacker, "Mobility: A Practical Guide to Managing Osteoarthritis and Falls," *Geriatrics* 58, no. 7 (2003): 22–29.

19. Messinger-Rapport and Thacker, "Mobility."

20. M. Vukojević, I. Soldo, and D. Granić, "Risk Factors Associated with Cerebral Palsy in Newborns," *Collegium Antropologicum* 33, supp. 2 (2009): 199–201; Jessica E. Miller et al., "Maternal Infections

during Pregnancy and Cerebral Palsy: A Population-Based Cohort Study," *Paediatric and Perinatal Epidemiology* 27, no. 6 (2013): 542–552, https://doi.org/10.1111/ppe.12082; and Hoda Z. Abdel-Hamid, "Cerebral Palsy," MedScape.com, August 12, 2016, retrieved September 12, 2017, http://emedicine. medscape.com/article/1179555-overview.

21. Abdel-Hamid, "Cerebral Palsy."

22. Susan M. Reid, John B. Carlin, and Dinah S. Reddihough, "Distribution of Motor Types in Cerebral Palsy: How Do Registry Data Compare?" *Developmental Medicine & Child Neurology* 53, no. 3 (2010): 233–238, https://doi.org/10.1111/j.1469-8749.2010.03844.x; and Abdel-Hamid, "Cerebral Palsy."

23. Abdel-Hamid, "Cerebral Palsy."

24. Mathew D. Sewell, Deborah M. Eastwood, and Neil Wimalasundera, "Managing Common Symptoms of Cerebral Palsy in Children," *The BMJ* 349, no. g5474 (2014): 27–31, https://doi.org/10.1136/bmj.g5474.

25. Abdel-Hamid, "Cerebral Palsy."

26. N. A. Murphy et al., "Costs and Complications of Hospitalizations for Children with Cerebral Palsy," *Pediatric Rehabilitation* 9, no. 1 (2006): 47–52, https://doi.org/10.1080/13638490500079476; Sewell, Eastwood, and Wimalasundera, "Managing Common Symptoms of Cerebral Palsy in Children"; and Abdel-Hamid, "Cerebral Palsy."

27. T. Schölderle et al., "Dysarthria in Adults with Cerebral Palsy: Clinical Presentation and Impacts on Communication," *Journal of Speech, Language, and Hearing Research* 59, no. 2 (2016), https://doi. org/10.1044/2015_JSLHR-S-15-0086.

28. Katherine C. Hustad et al., "Speech and Language Development in 2-Year-Old Children with Cerebral Palsy," *Developmental Neurorehabilitation* 17, no. 3 (2013): 167–175, https://doi. org/10.3109/17518423.2012.747009.

29. Schölderle et al., "Dysarthria in Adults with Cerebral Palsy."

30. Bronwyn Hemsley et al., "Supporting Communication for Children with Cerebral Palsy in Hospital: Views of Community and Hospital Staff," *Developmental Neurorehabilitation* 17, no. 3 (2014): 156–166, https://doi.org/10.3109/17518423.2012.741149.

31. Bronwyn Hemsley et al., "Parents and Children with Cerebral Palsy Discuss Communication Needs in Hospital, *Developmental Neurorehabilitation* 16, no. 6 (2013): 363–374, https://doi.org/10.3109/1751842 3.2012.758187.

32. Hemsley et al., "Parents and Children with Cerebral Palsy Discuss Communication Needs in Hospital," 366.

33. Hemsley et al., "Parents and Children with Cerebral Palsy Discuss Communication Needs in Hospital."

34. Hemsley et al., "Parents and Children with Cerebral Palsy Discuss Communication Needs in Hospital."

35. American Speech-Language-Hearing Association, "Augmentative and Alternative Communication (AAC)," http://www.asha.org/public/speech/disorders/AAC/.

36. Sewell, Eastwood, and Wimalasundera, "Managing Common Symptoms of Cerebral Palsy in Children."

37. N. A. Murphy et al., "Costs and Complications of Hospitalizations for Children with Cerebral Palsy"; and Sewell, Eastwood, and Wimalasundera, "Managing Common Symptoms of Cerebral Palsy."

38. Murphy et al., "Costs and Complications of Hospitalizations for Children with Cerebral Palsy."

39. Inmaculada Riquelme, Anna Zamorano, and Pedro Montoya, "Reduction of Pain Sensitivity after Somatosensory Therapy in Adults with Cerebral Palsy," *Frontiers in Human Neuroscience* 7 (2013): 1–7, https://doi.org/10.3389/fnhum.2013.00276.

40. T. L. Tewfik, "Cleft Lip and Palate and Mouth and Pharynx Deformities," MedScape.com, June 20, 2017, retrieved November 12, 2017, from https://emedicine.medscape.com/article/837347.

41. American Speech-Language-Hearing Association (ASHA), "Cleft Lip and Palate," retrieved April 3, 2018, from https://www.asha.org/Practice-Portal/Clinical-Topics/Cleft-Lip-and-Palate/.

42. Samantha E. Parker et al., "Updated National Birth Prevalence Estimates for Selected Birth Defects in the United States, 2004–2006," *Birth Defects Research Part A: Clinical and Molecular Teratology* 88, no. 12 (2010): 1,008–1,016, https://doi.org/10.1002/bdra.20735.

43. ASHA, "Cleft Lip and Palate."

44. American Cleft Palate-Craniofacial Association (ACPA), *Parameters for Evaluation and Treatment of Patients with Cleft Lip/Palate or Other Craniofacial Anomalies* (Chapel Hill, NC: ACPA, 2009).

45. Vanessa Martin and Sheila Greatrex-White, "An Evaluation of Factors Influencing Feeding in Babies with a Cleft Palate with and without a Cleft Lip," *Journal of Child Health Care* 18, no. 1 (2013): 72–83, https://doi.org/10.1177/1367493512473853; Linda Cooper-Brown et al., "Feeding and Swallowing Dysfunction in Genetic Syndromes," *Developmental Disabilities Research Reviews* 14, no. 2 (2008): 147–157, https://doi.org/10.1002/ddrr.19; and Gustaf Aniansson et al., "Otitis Media and Feeding with Breast Milk of Children with Cleft Palate," Scandinavian Journal of Plastic and Reconstructive Surgery and Hand Surgery 36, no. 1 (2002): 9–15, https://doi.org/10.1080/028443102753478318; and ASHA, "Cleft Lip and Palate."

46. I. Smillie et al., "Complications of Ventilation Tube Insertion in Children With and Without Cleft Palate: A Nested Case Control Comparison," *JAMA Otolaryngology–Head & Neck Surgery* 140, no. 10 (2014): 940–943, https://doi.org/10.1001/jamaoto.2014.1657; ACPA, *Parameters for Evaluation and Treatment of Patients with Cleft Lip/Palate or Other Craniofacial Anomalies*; and Aniansson et al., "Otitis Media and Feeding with Breast Milk of Children with Cleft Palate."

47. Aniansson et al., "Otitis Media and Feeding with Breast Milk of Children with Cleft Palate."

48. Tewfik, "Cleft Lip and Palate and Mouth and Pharynx Deformities."

49. Tewfik, "Cleft Lip and Palate and Mouth and Pharynx Deformities."

50. Isabelle Arteau-Gauthier, J. E. Leclerc, and A. Godbout, "Can We Predict a Difficult Intubation in Cleft Lip/Palate Patients?" *Journal of Otolaryngology-Head & Neck Surgery* 40, no. 5 (2011): 413–419; and F. S. Xue et al., "The Clinical Observation of Difficult Laryngoscopy and Difficult Intubation in Infants with Cleft Lip and Palate," *Pediatric Anesthesia* 16, no. 3 (2006): 283–289, https://doi.org/10.1111/j.1460-9592.2005.01762.x.

51. Xue et al., "Clinical Observation of Difficult Laryngoscopy and Difficult Intubation in Infants with Cleft Lip and Palate."

52. Little People of America, "Resources: Frequently Asked Questions," https://www.lpaonline.org/faq-.

53. "Dwarfism," MayoClinic.org, https://www.mayoclinic.org/diseases-conditions/dwarfism/symptoms-causes/syc-20371969.

54. Little People of America, "What Are the Most Common Types of Dwarfism?" http://www.lpaonline.org/faq-#Common.

55. G. Cabrera and B. Boling, *Achondroplasia* (Glendale, CA: Cinahl Information Systems, 2016).

56. Tracy L. Trotter and Judith G. Hall, "Health Supervision for Children with Achondroplasia," *Pediatrics* 116, no. 3 (2005): 771–783, https://doi.org/10.1542/peds.2005-1440.

57. Trotter and Hall, "Health Supervision for Children with Achondroplasia."

58. Nir Shimony et al., "Surgical Treatment for Cervicomedullary Compression among Infants with Achondroplasia," *Child's Nervous System* 31, no. 5 (2015): 743–750, https://doi.org/10.1007/s00381-015-2624-7; and Klaus Brühl et al., "Cerebral Spinal Fluid Flow, Venous Drainage and Spinal Cord Compression in Achondroplastic Children: Impact of Magnetic Resonance Findings for Decompressive Surgery at the Cranio-Cervical Junction," *European Journal of Pediatrics* 160, no. 1 (2001): 10–20, https://doi.org/10.1007/pl00008410.

59. Y. S. Hahn et al., "Paraplegia Resulting from Thoracolumbar Stenosis in a Seven-Month-Old Achondroplastic Dwarf," *Pediatric Neurosurgery* 15, no. 1 (1989): 39–43, https://doi.org/10.1159/000120439.

60. Kimberly E. Dessoffy, Peggy Modaff, and Richard M. Pauli, "Airway Malacia in Children with Achondroplasia," *American Journal of Medical Genetics Part A*, 164, no. 2 (2013): 407–414, https://doi.org/10.1002/ajmg.a.36303.

61. Shahla Afsharpaiman et al., "Respiratory Events and Obstructive Sleep Apnea in Children with Achondroplasia: Investigation and Treatment Outcomes," *Sleep and Breathing* 15, no. 4 (2011): 755–761, https://doi.org/10.1007/s11325-010-0432-6.

62. B. Schlüter et al., "Diagnostics and Management of Sleep-Related Respiratory Disturbances in Children with Skeletal Dysplasia Caused by FGFR3 Mutations (Achondroplasia and Hypochondroplasia)," *Georgian Medical News* 7–8, no. 196–197 (2011): 63–71.

63. Trotter and Hall, "Health Supervision for Children with Achondroplasia."

64. William O. Collins and Sukgi S. Choi, "Otolaryngologic Manifestations of Achondroplasia," *Archives of Otolaryngology–Head & Neck Surgery* 133, no. 3 (2007): 237–244, https://doi.org/10.1001/archotol.133.3.237.

65. Trotter and Hall, "Health Supervision for Children with Achondroplasia."

66. Trotter and Hall, "Health Supervision for Children with Achondroplasia."

67. Trotter and Hall, "Health Supervision for Children with Achondroplasia."

68. Celine Saint-Laurent et al., "Early Postnatal Soluble FGFR3 Therapy Prevents the Atypical Development of Obesity in Achondroplasia," *PLoS ONE* 13, no. 4 (2018): 1–18, https://doi.org/10.1371/journal.pone.0195876.

69. Özlem Taşoğlu et al., "Low Bone Density in Achondroplasia," *Clinical Rheumatology* 33, no. 5 (2014): 733–735, https://doi.org/10.1007/s10067-014-2577-3.

70. Kwang-Won Park et al., "Limb Lengthening in Patients with Achondroplasia," *Yonsei Medical Journal* 56, no. 6 (2015): 1,656–1,662, https://doi.org/10.3349/ymj.2015.56.6.1656.

71. Leslie M. Turner et al., "Spondyloepiphyseal Dysplasia Congenita," *Fetal and Pediatric Pathology* 29, no. 1 (2010): 57–62, https://doi.org/10.3109/15513810903266310; and US Department of Health and Human Services, National Institutes of Health, "Spondyloepiphyseal Dysplasia Congenita," US National Library of Medicine, Genetics Home Reference, April 2016, retrieved May 10, 2018, https://ghr.nlm.nih.gov/condition/spondyloepiphyseal-dysplasia-congenita.

72. US Department of Health and Human Services, National Institutes of Health, "Diastrophic Dysplasia," US National Library of Medicine, Genetics Home Reference, February 2008, retrieved May 10, 2018, https://ghr.nlm.nih.gov/condition/diastrophic-dysplasia; and Jonathan C. Honório et al., "Diastrophic Dysplasia: Prenatal Diagnosis and Review of the Literature," *São Paulo Medical Journal* 131, no. 2 (2013): 127–132, https://doi.org/10.1590/s1516-31802013000100024.

73. Trotter and Hall, "Health Supervision for Children with Achondroplasia."

74. US Department of Health and Human Services, National Institutes of Health, "Ehlers-Danlos Syndrome," US National Library of Medicine, Genetics Home Reference, https://ghr.nlm.nih.gov/condition/ehlers-danlos-syndrome.

75. J. Murray and M. Tyars, "A Case of Ehlers-Danlos Disease," *The British Medical Journal* 1, no. 1,415 (1940): 974, accessed from www.jstor.org/stable/20316755.

76. US Department of Health and Human Services, National Institutes of Health, "Ehlers-Danlos Syndrome," US National Library of Medicine, Genetics Home Reference, November 28, 2017, retrieved November 30, 2017, https://ghr.nlm.nih.gov/condition/ehlers-danlos-syndrome#statistics.

77. A. D. Nelson et al., "Ehlers Danlos Syndrome and Gastrointestinal Manifestations: A 20-Year Experience at Mayo Clinic," *Neurogastroenterology & Motility* 27 (2015): 1,657–1,666, https://doi.org/10.1111/nmo.12665.

78. Fransiska Malfait, Richard Wenstrup, and Anne De Paepe, "Classic Ehlers-Danlos Syndrome, Classic Type," August 18, 2011, retrieved December 12, 2017, https://www.ncbi.nlm.nih.gov/books/NBK1244/.

79. Nelson et al., "Ehlers Danlos Syndrome and Gastrointestinal Manifestations."

80. M. G. Pepin, M. L. Murray, and Peter H. Byers, "Vascular Ehlers-Danlos Syndrome," November 19, 2015, retrieved December 12, 2017, https://www.ncbi.nlm.nih.gov/books/NBK1494/.

81. Nelson et al., "Ehlers Danlos Syndrome and Gastrointestinal Manifestations."

82. Albert Busch et al., "Vascular Type Ehlers-Danlos Syndrome Is Associated with Platelet Dysfunction and Low Vitamin D Serum Concentration," *Orphanet Journal of Rare Diseases 11*, no. 1 (2016): 1–8, https://doi.org/10.1186/s13023-016-0491-2.

83. Xinyu Gui et al., "Systemic Multiple Aneurysms Caused by Vascular Ehlers-Danlos Syndrome," *Vascular and Endovascular Surgery* 50, no. 5 (2016): 354–358, https://doi.org/10.1177/1538574416647501.

84. Busch et al., "Vascular Type Ehlers-Danlos Syndrome."

85. Katsuhiko Hatake et al., "Respiratory Complications of Ehlers–Danlos Syndrome Type IV," *Legal Medicine* 15, no. 1 (2013): 23–27, https://doi.org/10.1016/j.legalmed.2012.07.005.

86. Mitzi L. Murray et al., "Pregnancy-Related Deaths and Complications in Women with Vascular Ehlers–Danlos Syndrome," *Genetics in Medicine* 16, no. 12 (2014): 874–880, https://doi.org/10.1038/gim.2014.53.

87. Sarah Soo-Hoo et al., "Ehlers-Danlos Syndrome Type IV: A Case Report," *Vascular and Endovascular Surgery* 50, no. 3 (2016): 156–159, https://doi.org/10.1177/1538574416627697.

88. Yael Gazit, Giris Jacob, and Rodney Grahame, "Ehlers-Danlos Syndrome—Hypermobility Type: A Much Neglected Multisystemic Disorder," *Rambam Maimonides Medical Journal* 7, no. 4 (2016): 1–10, https://doi.org/10.5041/rmmj.10261.

89. Claire Bovet, Matthew Carlson, and Matthew Taylor, "Quality of Life, Unmet Needs, and Iatrogenic Injuries in Rehabilitation of Patients with Ehlers-Danlos Syndrome Hypermobility Type/Joint Hypermobility Syndrome," *American Journal of Medical Genetics Part A*, 170, no. 8 (2016): 2,044–2,051, https://doi.org/10.1002/ajmg.a.37774.

90. Gazit, Jacob, and Grahame, "Ehlers-Danlos Syndrome—Hypermobility Type."

91. Justine Hugon-Rodin et al., "Gynecologic Symptoms and the Influence on Reproductive Life in 386 Women with Hypermobility Type Ehlers-Danlos Syndrome: A Cohort Study," Orphanet Journal of Rare Diseases 11, no. 124 (2016): 1–6, https://doi.org/10.1186/s13023-016-0511-2; Gazit, Jacob, and Grahame, "Ehlers-Danlos Syndrome—Hypermobility Type"; and Nelson et al., "Ehlers Danlos Syndrome and Gastrointestinal Manifestations."

92. Gazit, Jacob, and Grahame, "Ehlers-Danlos Syndrome—Hypermobility Type."

93. Bovet, Carlson, and Taylor, "Quality of Life, Unmet Needs, and Iatrogenic Injuries."

94. Brittney Murray et al., "Ehlers-Danlos Syndrome, Hypermobility Type: A Characterization of the Patients' Lived Experience," *American Journal of Medical Genetics Part A*, 161, no. 12 (2013): 2, 981–2,988, https://doi.org/10.1002/ajmg.a.36293.

95. Soo-Hoo et al., "Ehlers-Danlos Syndrome Type IV."

96. Justin E. Sam and Mala Dharmalingam, "Osteogenesis Imperfecta," *Indian Journal of Endocrinology and Metabolism*, 21, no. 6 (2017): 903, https://doi.org/10.4103/ijem.ijem_220_17.

97. Sam and Dharmalingam, "Osteogenesis Imperfecta."

98. US Department of Health and Human Services, National Institutes of Health, "Osteogenesis Imperfecta Overview," Osteoporosis and Related Bone Diseases National Resource Center, May 2015, Publication No. 15–AR–8004, retrieved December 31, 2017, https://www.bones.nih.gov/sites/bones/files/overview_oi.pdf.

99. Osteogenesis Imperfecta Foundation, "Types of OI," 2015, retrieved December 31, 2017, http://www.oif.org/site/PageServer?pagename=AOI_Types.

100. Nadja Fratzl-Zelman et al., "Classification of Osteogenesis Imperfecta," *Wiener Medizinische Wochenschrift* 165, no. 13–14 (2015): 264–270, https://doi.org/10.1007/s10354-015-0368-3.

101. Inas H. Thomas and Linda A. DiMeglio, "Advances in the Classification and Treatment of Osteogenesis Imperfecta," *Current Osteoporosis Reports* 14, no. 1 (2016): 1–9, https://doi.org/10.1007/s11914-016-0299-y.

102. Ronit Marom et al., "Pharmacological and Biological Therapeutic Strategies for Osteogenesis Imperfecta," American Journal of Medical Genetics, Part C: Seminars in *Medical Genetics*, 172, no. 4 (2016): 367–383, https://doi.org/10.1002/ajmg.c.31532.

103. A. Forlino and J. C. Marini, "Osteogenesis Imperfecta," *Lancet* 387, no. 10,028 (2016): 1,657–1,671, doi:10.1016/s0140-6736(15)00728-x; Thomas and Dimeglio, "Advances in the Classification and Treatment of Osteogenesis Imperfecta"; and Heike Hoyer-Kuhn, Christian Netzer, and Oliver Semler, "Osteogenesis Imperfecta: Pathophysiology and Treatment," *Wiener Medizinische Wochenschrift* 165, no. 13–14 (2015): 278–284, https://doi.org/10.1007/s10354-015-0361-x.

104. Forlino and Marini, "Osteogenesis Imperfecta"; Hoyer-Kuhn, Netzer, and Semler, "Osteogenesis Imperfecta: Pathophysiology and Treatment."

105. Thomas and DiMeglio, "Advances in the Classification and Treatment of Osteogenesis Imperfecta."

106. Elaine M. Pereira, "Clinical Perspectives on Osteogenesis Imperfecta versus Non-Accidental Injury," *American Journal of Medical Genetics, Part C: Seminars in Medical Genetics*, 169, no. 4 (2015): 302–306, https://doi.org/10.1002/ajmg.c.31463.

107. Pereira, "Clinical Perspectives on Osteogenesis Imperfecta versus Non-Accidental Injury."

108. Pereira, "Clinical Perspectives on Osteogenesis Imperfecta versus Non-Accidental Injury."

109. K. Golshani et al., "Osteogenesis Imperfecta," *Delaware Medical Journal* 88, no. 6 (2016): 178–185.

110. Forlino and Marini, "Osteogenesis Imperfecta"; Thomas and DiMeglio, "Advances in the Classification and Treatment of Osteogenesis Imperfecta"; and Golshani et al., "Osteogenesis Imperfecta."

111. Thomas and DiMeglio, "Advances in the Classification and Treatment of Osteogenesis Imperfecta"; and Golshani et al., "Osteogenesis Imperfecta."

112. Thomas and DiMeglio, "Advances in the Classification and Treatment of Osteogenesis Imperfecta."

113. US Department of Health and Human Services, Centers for Disease Control and Prevention, "Statistics on Spina Bifida," https://www.cdc.gov/ncbddd/spinabifida/data.html.

114. Mark R. Foster and Kat Kolaski, "Spina Bifida," MedScape.com, September 22, 2016, retrieved August 29, 2017, http://emedicine.medscape.com/article/311113-overview#a2.

115. L. Werhagen et al., "Medical Complications in Adults with Spina Bifida," *Clinical Neurology and Neurosurgery* 115, no. 8 (2013): 1,226–1,229, https://doi.org/10.1016/j.clineuro.2012.11.014.

116. Samantha E. Parker et al., "A Description of Spina Bifida Cases and Co-occurring Malformations, 1976–2011," *American Journal of Medical Genetics*, Part A,164A, no. 2, (2014): 432–440, https://doi.org/10.1002/ajmg.a.36324; and Foster and Kolaski, "Spina Bifida."

117. Seyhmus K. Özel and Ibrahim Ulman, "Contemporary Urological Management of Spina Bifida," *Journal of Pediatric Research in Pediatric Endocrinology* 3, no. 4 (2016): 168–174, https://doi.org/10.4274/jpr.33154.

118. Linda Cooper-Brown et al., "Feeding and Swallowing Dysfunction in Genetic Syndromes," *Developmental Disabilities Research Reviews* 14, no. 2 (2008): 154, https://doi.org/10.1002/ddrr.19.

119. US Department of Health and Human Services, National Institutes of Health, National Institute of Neurological Disorders and Stroke, "Chiari Malformation Fact Sheet," 2017, retrieved November 28, 2017, https://www.ninds.nih.gov/Disorders/Patient-Caregiver-Education/Fact-Sheets/Chiari-Malformation-Fact-Sheet.

120. Michael D. Jenkinson et al., "Cognitive and Functional Outcome in Spina Bifida-Chiari II Malformation," *Child's Nervous System* 27, no. 6 (2011): 967–974, https://doi.org/10.1007/s00381-010-1368-7.

121. Kimiaki Hashiguchi et al., "Sequential Morphological Change of Chiari Malformation Type II Following Surgical Repair of Myelomeningocele," *Child's Nervous System* 32, no. 6 (2016): 1,069–1,078, https://doi.org/10.1007/s00381-016-3041-2; Jenkinson et al., "Cognitive and Functional Outcome in Spina Bifida-Chiari II Malformation"; Jenifer Juranek and Michael. S. Salman, "Anomalous Development of Brain Structure and Function in Spina Bifida Myelomeningocele," *Developmental Disabilities Research Reviews* 16, no. 1 (2010): 23–30, https://doi.org/10.1002/ddrr.88; and Cooper-Brown et al., "Feeding and Swallowing Dysfunction in Genetic Syndromes," 147–157.

122. Hashiguchi et al., "Sequential Morphological Change of Chiari Malformation Type II Following Surgical Repair of Myelomeningocele."

123. Werhagen et al., "Medical Complications in Adults with Spina Bifida"; and Melissa A. Matson, E. Mark Mahone, and T. Andrew Zabel, "Serial Neuropsychological Assessment and Evidence of Shunt Malfunction in Spina Bifida: A Longitudinal Case Study," *Child Neuropsychology* 11, no. 4 (2005): 315–332, https://doi.org/10.1080/09297040490916910.

124. Todd C. Hankinson, "Ventriculoatrial Shunt Placement," MedScape.com, March 11, 2016, retrieved August 18, 2017, from http://emedicine.medscape.com/article/1895753-overview#a1.

125. A. Khalil et al., "Prenatal Prediction of Need for Ventriculoperitoneal Shunt in Open Spina Bifida," Ultrasound in Obstetrics and Gynecology 43, no. 2 (2014): 159–164, https://doi.org/10.1002/uog.13202.

126. P. Tomlinson and I. D. Sugarman, "Complications with Shunts in Adults with Spina Bifida," *BMJ* 311, no. 7,000 (1995): 286–287, https://doi.org/10.1136/bmj.311.7000.286.

127. Theodosios Birbilis et al., "Spontaneous Bowel Perforation Complicating Ventriculoperitoneal Shunt: A Case Report," *Cases Journal* 2, no. 1 (2009): 8,251–8,255, https://doi.org/10.4076/1757-1626-2-8251; and Atsumi Tamura, Dai Shida, and Kyosuke Tsutsumi, "Abdominal Cerebrospinal Fluid Pseudocyst Occurring 21 Years after Ventriculoperitoneal Shunt Placement: A Case Report," *BMC Surgery* 13, no. 1 (2013), 1–4, https://doi.org/10.1186/1471-2482-13-27.

128. T. Michael et al., "Risk Factors for Latex Allergy in Patients with Spina Bifida," *Clinical and Experimental Allergy* 26, no. 8 (1996): 934–939, https://doi.org/10.1111/j.1365-2222.1996.tb00629.x; and Foster and Kolaski, "Spina Bifida."

129. Dietke Buck et al., "Ventricular Shunts and the Prevalence of Sensitization and Clinically Relevant Allergy to Latex in Patients with Spina Bifida," *Pediatric Allergy and Immunology* 11, no. 2 (2000): 111–115, https://doi.org/10.1034/j.1399-3038.2000.00039.x; and E. Ausili et al., "Prevalence of Latex Allergy in Spina Bifida: Genetic and Environmental Factors," European Review for Medical and Pharmacological Sciences 11, no. 3 (2007): 149–153.

130. T. Eiwegger et al., "Early Exposure to Latex Products Mediates Latex Sensitization in Spina Bifida but Not in Other Diseases with Comparable Latex Exposure Rates," *Clinical Experimental Allergy* 36, no. 10 (2006): 1,244, https://doi.org/10.1111/j.1365-2222.2006.02564.x, 1,244.

131. Katharina Blumchen et al., "Effects of Latex Avoidance on Latex Sensitization, Atopy and Allergic Diseases in Patients with Spina Bifida," *Allergy* 65 no. 12 (2010): 1,585–1593, https://doi.org/10.1111/j.1398-9995.2010.02447.x.

132. Blumchen et al., "Effects of Latex Avoidance on Latex Sensitization, Atopy and Allergic Diseases in Patients with Spina Bifida,"; Ausili et al., "Prevalence of Latex Allergy in Spina Bifida: Genetic and Environmental Factors"; A. Nieto et al., "The Search of Latex Sensitization in Spina Bifida: Diagnostic Approach," *Clinical and Experimental Allergy* 30, no. 2 (2000): 264–269, https://doi.org/10.1046/j.1365-2222.2000.00705.x; Michael et al., "Risk Factors for Latex Allergy in Patients with Spina Bifida."

133. Miaozong Wu, James Mcintosh, and Jian Liu, "Current Prevalence Rate of Latex Allergy: Why It Remains A Problem," *Journal of Occupational Health* 58, no. 2 (2016): 138–144, https://doi.org/10.1539/joh.15-0275-ra.

134. "Home page," Spina Bifida Association, http://spinabifidaassociation.org/wp-content/uploads/2015/07/latex-in-the-home-and-community-eng.pdf.

135. Wu, Mcintosh, and Liu, "Current Prevalence Rate of Latex Allergy: Why It Remains a Problem"; and D. H. Beezhold et al., "Latex Allergy Can Induce Clinical Reactions to Specific Foods," *Clinical and Experimental Allergy* 26, no. 4 (1996): 416–422, https://doi.org/10.1111/j.1365-2222.1996.tb00557.x.

136. Foster and Kolaski, "Spina Bifida"; Özel and Ulman, "Contemporary Urological Management of Spina Bifida"; and Werhagen et al., "Medical Complications in Adults with Spina Bifida."

137. Subramanian Vaidyanathan et al., "Pyonephrosis and Urosepsis in a 41-Year-Old Patient with Spina Bifida: Case Report of a Preventable Death," *Patient Safety in Surgery* 6, no. 10 (2012): 1–8, https://doi.org/10.1186/1754-9493-6-10.

138. Foster and Kolaski, "Spina Bifida."

139. Katherine Ottolini et al., "Wound Care Challenges in Children and Adults with Spina Bifida: An Open-Cohort Study," *Journal of Pediatric Rehabilitation Medicine: An Interdisciplinary Approach* 6, no. 1 (2013): 1–10, https://doi.org/10.3233/PRM-130231.

140. M. Porter and J. Kelly, "Pressure Ulcer Treatment in a Patient with Spina Bifida," *Nursing Standard* 28, no. 35 (2014): 60–69.

141. Elizabeth A. Szalay and Asad Cheema, "Children with Spina Bifida Are at Risk for Low Bone Density," *Clinical Orthopaedics and Related Research* 469, no. 5 (2010): 1,253–1,257, https://doi.org/10.1007/s11999-010-1634-8; V. Martinelli et al., "Risk of Fracture Prevention in Spina Bifida Patients: Correlation between Bone Mineral Density, Vitamin D, and Electrolyte Values," *Child's Nervous System* 31, no. 8 (2015): 1,361–1,365, https://doi.org/10.1007/s00381-015-2726-2; and Foster and Kolaski, "Spina Bifida."

142. Minn M. Soe et al., "Health Risk Behaviors among Young Adults with Spina Bifida," *Developmental Medicine & Child Neurology* 54, no. 11 (2012): 1,057–1,064, https://doi.org/10.1111/j.1469-8749.2012.04402.x.

143. Gregory S. Liptak and Ahmad El Samra, "Optimizing Health Care for Children with Spina Bifida," *Developmental Disabilities Research Review*, Special Issue: Spina Bifida—A Multidisciplinary Perspective, 16, no. 1 (2010): 66–75, https://doi.org/10.1002/ddrr.91.

144. Soe et al., "Health Risk Behaviors among Young Adults with Spina Bifida."

145. Beverly Petterson et al. "Co-occurrence of Birth Defects and Intellectual Disability," *Paediatric and Perinatal Epidemiology* 21, no. 1 (2007): 65–75, htttps://doi.org/10.1111/j.1365-3016.2007.00774.x.

146. Foster and Kolaski, "Spina Bifida."

147. Cooper-Brown et al., "Feeding and Swallowing Dysfunction in Genetic Syndromes"; Thomas S. Webb, "Optimizing Health Care for Adults with Spina Bifida," *Developmental Disabilities Research Reviews* 16, no. 1 (2010): 76–81, https://doi.org/10.1002/ddrr.99; and Foster and Kolaski, "Spina Bifida."

148. Brian S. Amour et al., "Prevalence and Causes of Paralysis—United States, 2013," *American Journal of Public Health* 106, no. 10 (2016): 1,855–1,857.

149. National Spinal Cord Injury Statistical Center, *Spinal Cord Injuries: Facts and Figures at a Glance* (Birmingham, AL: University of Alabama at Birmingham, 2015), https://www.nscisc.uab.edu/Public/Facts%202015%20Aug.pdf.

150. Lawrence S. Chin, "Spinal Cord Injuries," MedScape.com, August 10, 2017, retrieved December 19, 2017, https://emedicine.medscape.com/article/793582-overview.

151. Michael Abraham, Jason Brown, and Andrew D. Perron, "Spinal Cord Injury," *Trauma Reports* 17, no. 6 (2016): 1–15, https://www.ahcmedia.com/articles/139075-spinal-cord-injury.

152. American Spinal Injury Association (ASIA) and the International Spinal Cord Society (ISCS), "ASIA Impairment Scale," *International Standards for Neurological Classification of Spinal Cord Injury* (ASIA and ISCS, November 2015), http://asia-spinalinjury.org/wp-content/uploads/2016/02/International_Stds_Diagram_Worksheet.pdf.

153. Chin, "Spinal Cord Injuries."

154. E. M. Hagen et al., "Cardiovascular and Urological Dysfunction in Spinal Cord Injury," Acta Neurologica Scandinavica 124 (2011): 71–78, https://doi.org/10.1111/j.1600-0404.2011.01547.x.

155. E. J. McGuire, "Urologic Care of the Spinal Cord Injury Patient," *Urology Times* (December 2009): S4–S10.

156. Jacqueline Cragg and Andrei Krassioukov, "Five Things to Know about Autonomic Dysreflexia," *Canadian Medical Association Journal* 184, no. 1 (2012): 66, https://doi.org/10.1503/cmaj.110859.

157. Andrei Krassioukov et al., "A Systematic Review of the Management of Autonomic Dysreflexia Following Spinal Cord Injury," *Archives of Physical Medicine and Rehabilitation* 90, no. 4 (2009): 682–695, https://doi.org/10.1016/j.apmr.2008.10.017; and Hagen et al., "Cardiovascular and Urological Dysfunction in Spinal Cord Injury."

158. Huseyin Gunduz and Duygu F. Binak, "Autonomic Dysreflexia: An Important Cardiovascular Complication in Spinal Cord Injury Patients," *Cardiology Journal* 19, no. 2 (2012): 215–219, accessible from https://doi.org/10.5603/cj.2012.0040.

159. Darryl Wan and Andrei V. Krassioukov, "Life-Threatening Outcomes Associated with Autonomic Dysreflexia: A Clinical Review," *Journal of Spinal Cord Medicine* 37, no. 1 (2013): 2–10, https://doi.org/10.1179/2045772313y.0000000098; Cragg and Krassioukov, "Five Things to Know about Autonomic Dysreflexia"; Gunduz and Binak, "Autonomic Dysreflexia: An Important Cardiovascular Complication in Spinal Cord Injury Patients"; Hagen et al., "Cardiovascular and Urological Dysfunction in Spinal Cord Injury"; Krassioukov et al., "A Systematic Review of the Management of Autonomic Dysreflexia Following Spinal Cord Injury"; and Ryan O. Stephenson and Jeffrey Berliner, "Autonomic Dysreflexia in Spinal Cord Injury: Overview, Pathophysiology, Causes of Autonomic Dysreflexia," MedScape.com, May 16, 2018, retrieved July 3, 2018, https://emedicine.medscape.com/article/322809-overview#a1.

160. Jiri Kriz, Ross Andel, and Renata Hakova, "Delayed Diagnosis of an Unsuspected Pelvic Fracture in a Patient with Tetraplegia," *Journal of Spinal Cord Medicine* 37, no. 4 (2014): 425–428, https://doi.org/10.1179/2045772313y.0000000178.

161. Krassioukov et al., "A Systematic Review of the Management of Autonomic Dysreflexia Following Spinal Cord Injury"; Hagen et al., "Cardiovascular and Urological Dysfunction in Spinal Cord Injury"; Gunduz and Binak, "Autonomic Dysreflexia: An Important Cardiovascular Complication in Spinal Cord Injury Patients"; and Jordan W. Squair et al., "Emergency Management of Autonomic Dysreflexia with Neurologic Complications," *Canadian Medical Association Journal* 188, no. 15 (2016): 1,100–1,103, https://doi.org/10.1503/cmaj.151311.

162. S. Matsumoto et al., "Prospective Study of Deep Vein Thrombosis in Patients with Spinal Cord Injury Not Receiving Anticoagulant Therapy," *Spinal Cord* 53, no. 4 (2015): 306–309, https://doi.org/10.1038/sc.2015.4.

163. Hilal Onmez et al., "Bilateral Upper-Extremity Deep Vein Thrombosis Following Central Cord Syndrome," *Journal of Spinal Cord Medicine* 36, no. 3 (2013): 243–246, https://doi.org/10.1179/2045772 313y.0000000096.

164. McGuire, "Urologic Care of the Spinal Cord Injury Patient," s6.

165. Hagen et al., "Cardiovascular and Urological Dysfunction in Spinal Cord Injury,"

166. Jelena Svircev, "Osteoporosis and Fractures in Persons with SCI: What, Why, and How to Manage" (Power-Point presentation, Spinal Cord Injury Forum, Department of Veterans Affairs, Puget Sound Health Care System, November 13, 2012, retrieved November 19, 2017, http://sci.washington.edu/info/ forums/reports/osteoporosis.asp.

167. Svircev, "Osteoporosis and Fractures in Persons with SCI."

168. Tiffiny Carlson, "How to Greet Someone in a Wheelchair," March 2, 2018, retrieved March 3, 2018, https://www.spinalcord.com/blog/how-to-greet-someone-in-a-wheelchair.

6

Mental Health Disorders

You are en route to a psychiatric emergency call for a 45-year-old man. Dispatch reports the patient is combative, but the police have arrived and secured the scene, so you proceed in. You are met in the front yard by an officer who tells you that 911 was called by the neighbor who initially found the patient, Brian, in the front yard, babbling and confused. When the neighbor approached him to see what was wrong, he began cursing and swatting at her. The officer says, "I don't know what's wrong, but he's nuts." He follows you and your partner into the house where Brian, in the company of additional officers, is pacing and yelling. An officer hands you two prescription bottles containing anti-depressant and anti-anxiety medications and says, "He's gone off his rocker." You speak calmly to Brian and ask him if you can conduct an assessment and check his blood sugar. He reluctantly agrees. The blood glucose monitor reads 37mg/dL, which is very low. Although Brian apparently has at least one mental health diagnosis based on the medications in the house, he also has diabetes, which the police did not discover as his insulin was in the refrigerator. You administer oral glucose paste while your partner draws up some glucagon. In a few minutes, Brian is oriented and calm and agrees to transport to the hospital for additional care.

According to the National Institute of Mental Health, almost 45 million people in the United States, or 1 in 6 adults (18%), live with mental illness.[1] Mental illness is defined as any mental, behavioral, or emotional disorder, with severity ranging from mild to severe. These disorders include anxiety, depression, post-traumatic stress disorder, bipolar disorder, obsessive-compulsive disorder, schizophrenia, and many others. Individuals with mental health issues are at greater risk for substance abuse, homelessness, and chronic health issues.[2] It is likely that as a prehospital provider you will encounter individuals with all ranges and types of mental health issues. This chapter will provide some general guidance for communicating with and assessing patients with mental health concerns, including a discussion on physical illnesses that may look like, or mimic, a psychiatric problem, and/or have comorbid physical symptoms with a psychiatric problem.

Communication with people who have mental illness

You may be concerned about interacting with and communicating effectively with someone living with mental illness. This is understandable, as mental health issues are often stigmatized in our society, and those who live with mental illness are often portrayed as unstable, violent, or dangerous. And while that can certainly be the case, most people with mental illness present no danger to others.

When speaking with and assessing someone with a mental illness, here are some suggestions for facilitating communication:[3]

- Be respectful.
- Stay calm even if they are not.
- Ask questions to clarify your understanding, e.g., "Let me see if I have this right. You had difficulty breathing after fighting with your sister, but you are better now."
- Find areas you can agree on, e.g., "We both agree that your pain is severe."
- Give them time to process your questions and to respond.
- Do not interrupt, criticize, or tell them what to do or believe.
- If your patient is hallucinating or delusional, acknowledge that their hallucinations are real to them but do not pretend that you see or hear their hallucinations, e.g., "Yes, I imagine that seeing vampires is very frightening."
- Give them personal space, especially if they are agitated or frightened.
- Do not lie to them to get them to agree to something.
- Set limits for conversations that are going nowhere or becoming cyclical, e.g., "I see that you have more to say, but it is time to get in the ambulance to go to the hospital."
- Call for help if the situation deteriorates. Your personal safety is paramount.

When a physical condition mimics a mental health disorder

When assessing patients with an apparent mental health crisis, it is important to remember that there are some physical conditions that can mimic mental illnesses, and/or cause anxiety, depression, panic, or other psychiatric symptoms.

Hentz[4] and Hedaya[5] provide some general considerations for assessing patients with possible mental health issues and when to consider that a physical medical condition might be mimicking or hiding a psychiatric condition:

- A new onset of psychiatric symptoms with no personal history or relevant triggering event.

- A late-in-age new onset of symptoms, for example, an elderly person with a panic attack and no previous history of anxiety.

- A new onset of symptoms that emerge with a headache, loss of neurologic or cognitive function, unusual feelings or sensations such as tingling, disconnection to one's self (dissociation), or hallucinations. One example might be an elderly person with no previous diagnosis of dementia who is experiencing altered mentation.

- Any drug use, including prescribed, illicit, or over-the-counter drugs, vitamins, or herbal supplements, should be considered as a cause of symptoms.

While there may be very little you can do for some of these issues in the prehospital setting, it is still important to conduct a thorough assessment in order to identify any issue that you can treat in the field. Prehospital providers also play an important role in potentially reducing the time to a definitive diagnosis in the emergency department by not assuming all psychiatric symptoms are caused by mental illness. Conducting a thorough physical exam and taking a complete history can help you find additional signs and symptoms that may differentiate between a true psychiatric emergency and a "medical mimic." Of course, our job is not to reach a definitive diagnosis in the field, but to gather as much information as possible to address the immediate emergency and to provide comprehensive information to the receiving physician at the emergency department.

Psychiatrist Robert Hedaya developed a mnemonic to help providers remember the major categories of potential medical mimics: **THINC MED**.[6]

T—Tumors

Tumors in any part of the body can cause physical symptoms, including pain, but they also can cause a myriad of psychiatric and emotional disturbances:

- Brain tumors can cause memory loss and personality and mood changes.[7]
- Pancreatic tumors can cause depression.[8]
- Adrenal gland tumors can cause panic attacks.[9]

H—Hormones

An increase, descrease, or absence of hormones can lead to emotional disturbances:

- Hypothyroidism can lead to fatigue and depression.[10]
- Hyperthyroidism can cause anxiety, depression, mania, and psychosis.[11]
- Too much cortisol from the adrenal glands (Cushing's disease) can cause anxiety, depression, mania, and irritability.[12]
- Too little cortisol (Addison's disease) can cause depression, personality changes, memory loss, and irritability.[13]
- Too much insulin causes hypoglycemia, leading to anxiety, aggression, distractibility, irritability, and confusion.[14]
- Too little insulin causes hyperglycemia, leading to lethargy (which can look like depression) and tachycardia (which can look like anxiety).[15]

I—Infectious and immune disease

- Strep infections can lead to tics and obsessive-compulsive behaviors.[16]
- Lupus can lead to cognitive deficits, depression, and anxiety.[17]
- Urinary tract infections, especially in the elderly, can cause confusion and memory loss.[18]

N—Nutrition

- Vitamin B-12 (*colbalamin*) deficiency can cause dementia, mood disorders, paranoia, hallucinations, and panic attacks.[19]

- Vitamin B-1 (*thiamine*) deficiency (common in chronic alcohol abuse) can cause dementia, fatigue, apathy (mimics depression), and psychosis.[20]
- Vitamin B-6 (*pyridoxine*) deficiency is related to depression, confusion, irritability, cognitive deficits, and dementia in the elderly.[21]

C—Central nervous system

- Traumatic brain injury can lead to confusion, aggression, and disorientation.[22]
- Seizures can cause unusual sensations (which could be misinterpreted as psychosis or hallucinations), rage, and irritability, especially in the postictal state.
- The motor slowing and decrease in facial expression associated with Parkinson's disease can be misinterpreted as depression or apathy.[23]

M—Miscellaneous

- Sleep apnea causes interrupted sleep and lowered SpO_2 during sleep, which can lead to fatigue and depression.
- Anemia can cause decreased oxygen delivery to the body's tissues leading to fatigue, heart palpitations, and trouble breathing, which can look like depression or anxiety.

E—Electrolyte imbalances and environmental toxins

- *Electrolytes* are substances within the body that conduct electrical impulses between cells. They are necessary for a myriad of body functions such as muscle contraction, nerve function, and blood pressure. Electrolytes include the following:
    - Sodium
    - Potassium
    - Calcium
    - Bicarbonate
    - Magnesium
    - Chloride
    - Phosphate

- When an electrolyte becomes unbalanced, either too high or too low, it can cause multiple symptoms, including confusion, irritability, dementia, mood changes, and fatigue.[24]

- Exposure to environmental toxins can impact a patient's mental status. The effects are dependent on the toxin, length of exposure, and many other factors. This exposure may be deliberate (self-harm or suicide attempt) or accidental (workplace exposure or accidental spill).

D—Drugs

- Be sure to consider the ingestion of any substance, including prescribed medications, over-the-counter medications, illicit drugs, vitamins, dietary supplements, etc. when assessing a patient with an unusual onset of psychiatric symptoms.

- There could be a new onset of allergy or sensitivity to a medication, or an interaction with something newly prescribed or ingested and an established medication.

- An increase in dose or increases in ingestion can cause new symptoms. For example, a significant caffeine increase can cause restlessness, anxiety, and irritability.

ADHD

A 32-year-old woman calls 911 for difficulty breathing. You arrive on scene and find the patient, Sara, lying on the couch, breathing shallowly and rapidly. She reports a history of anxiety and says she felt the onset of a panic attack. Instead of taking her anxiety medication, Sara accidentally took two of her daughter's Adderall capsules. She is now feeling severely anxious and agitated, as well as tachypneic and tachycardic. You place Sara on the cardiac monitor and capnography to monitor her vital signs, call medical control for orders for activated charcoal, and transport her to the ED for assessment and observation.

Attention deficit/hyperactivity disorder (ADHD) is a cluster of symptoms that manifest with difficulties with attention, hyperactivity, and impulsivity. The APA[25] provides the diagnostic criteria for ADHD, which can be diagnosed by a psychiatrist, clinical psychologist, or developmental pediatrician, or through school evaluations.

Individuals can be identified in three ways:

- Predominantly inattentive
- Predominantly hyperactive/impulsive
- Combined (has symptoms of both inattention and hyperactivity/impulsivity)

ADHD has two broad categories of symptoms required for diagnosis.[26]

1. A persistent pattern of *inattention* that includes behaviors such as the following:
   - Failure to pay close attention to details required for work completion
   - Making careless mistakes
   - Having difficulty sustaining attention, maintaining focus, and following through on tasks
   - Appearing frequently distracted and sidetracked
   - Having difficulty organizing tasks and belongings
   - Losing or misplacing belongings or needed materials
   - Avoiding work that requires focused attention
   - Being forgetful

2. A persistent pattern of *impulsivity* and *hyperactivity* that includes behaviors such as the following:
   - Fidgeting or squirming frequently
   - Leaving seat when expected to remain seated
   - Running or climbing on things in situations where it is inappropriate
   - Feeling restless
   - Difficulty playing or engaging in quiet activities
   - Appearing "motor-driven" or always moving
   - Talking excessively and out of turn
   - Difficulty waiting
   - Interrupting others' conversations or activities
   - Using others' belongings without permission

In addition to meeting the specific criteria, the symptoms must have manifested themselves before the age of 12 years (although the diagnosis itself is not required before 12 years of age), must have persisted for at least six months, and must interfere with school, work, and social activities.[27] The APA estimates ADHD occurs in 5% of children and 2.5% of adults.[28] ADHD is frequently comorbid with many other mental health conditions such as the following:

- Oppositional defiant disorder
  - 25% of children with inattentive ADHD
  - 50% of children with combined ADHD

- Conduct disorder
  - 25% of children with combined ADHD

- Disruptive mood dysregulation disorder
- Specific learning disorder
- Anxiety disorders and major depressive disorder
- Intermittent explosive disorder
- Personality disorders
- Obsessive-compulsive disorder
- Tic disorders
- Autism spectrum disorder

Conway et al. also note that children with ADHD experience higher rates of attachment trauma such as foster care placement, sexual abuse, and overall maltreatment.[29]

Although ADHD is not likely to precipitate an EMS response by itself, it is still a frequent reason behind emergency department visits by children, although many are avoidable and may be more appropriately addressed by a primary care physician.[30] Lynch et al. reported in their study of 28,000 behavior-related emergency department visits by children with Medicaid that 24% were for ADHD-related care, and 97% of those children were discharged home from the emergency department.[31] The reasons for the visits included poisoning, injuries, vague respiratory and gastrointestinal complaints, and ADHD-related concerns. The authors concluded that many families are using the emergency department as "a primary care mental health service delivery setting."[32] This is due in part to inadequate mental health resources.

Medication for ADHD

The biggest concerns surrounding pharmaceutical treatments of ADHD are their side effects and the potential for abuse, overdose, and addiction.

Several classes of medication are used to treat ADHD, including short- and long-acting stimulants, nonstimulants, and antidepressants. Table 6–1 lists the classes of medications and some examples, along with their side effects.

Table 6–1. Classes of medications

Classes of Medications				
Class	Generic name	Medication name	Non-ADHD uses	Reported side effects
Stimulants	Methylphenidate HCl	Ritalin Concerta Metadate	Narcolepsy	• Weight loss • Poor appetite • Growth delay • Sleeplessness • Irritability • Tics • Cardiac problems • Hypertension • Increased psychiatric problems
	Dextroamphetamine Sulf-Saccharate	Adderall	Narcolepsy	• Headache • Sleeplessness • Irritability • Dry mouth • Loss of appetite • Cardiovascular problems • Sudden death in people with previous cardiac problems
	Dextroamphetamine Sulfate	Dexedrine	Narcolepsy	• Headache • Sleeplessness • Irritability • Dry mouth • Loss of appetite • Cardiovascular problems • Sudden death in people with previous cardiac problems

Table 6–1. ...*continued*

	Amphetamine Sulfate	Evekeo	Narcolepsy Obesity	• Tachycardia • Hypertension • Restlessness • Tics • Diarrhea • Constipation • Weight loss • Loss of appetite
	Dexmethyl-phenidate HCl	Focalin		• Headache • Sleeplessness • Irritability • Dry mouth • Loss of appetite • Cardiovascular problems • Sudden death in people with previous cardiac problems
	Lisdexam-fetamine Dimesylate	Vyvanse	Binge eating disorder	• Headache • Sleeplessness • Irritability • Dry mouth • Loss of appetite • Cardiovascular problems • Sudden death in people with previous cardiac problems
Non-stimulants	Clonidine	Catapres	Hypertension Hot flashes Excessive sweating	• Hypotension • Rebound hypertension if stopped suddenly • Fatigue • Dry mouth • Constipation • Diarrhea • Headache • Fever • Cold-like symptoms

Table 6–1. ...*continued*

	Guanfacine HCl	Intuniv Tenex	Hypertension	• Sleepiness • Headache • Fatigue • Dizziness • Abdominal pain • Weight gain
	Atomoxetine HCl	Strattera		• Sleep problems • Anxiety • Fatigue • Upset stomach • Dizziness • Dry mouth. • Liver damage (rarely) • Suicidal ideation
Antide-pressants	Imipramine HCl	Tofranil	Depression Bed wetting	• Anxiety • Fatigue • Upset stomach • Dizziness • Dry mouth • Heart dysrhythmias • Breast swelling • Blurred vision • Suicidal ideation
	Bupropion HCl	Wellbutrin	Anxiety Depression Obsessive-compulsive disorder Weight loss Smoking cessation	• Headache • Seizures • Sore throat • Muscle pain • Weight loss or gain • Suicidal ideation

Sources: Samuele Cortese et al., "Practitioner Review: Current Best Practice in the Management of Adverse Events during Treatment with ADHD Medications in Children and Adolescents," *Journal of Child Psychology and Psychiatry* 54, no. 3 (2013): 227–246, https://doi.org/10.1111/jcpp.12036; "ADHD: Treatment and Care," WebMD, https://www.webmd.com/add-adhd/guide/adhd-medication-chart#1; and "ADHD Drugs," RxList, https://www.rxlist.com/.

ADHD Concerns That Might Precipitate an EMS Response

Overdose

Individuals taking any medication can potentially overdose, either accidentally or deliberately. Follow your local protocols for overdose and consider calling a poison control center for guidance on the use of activated charcoal or a specific antidote if allowed by protocols.

Substance abuse

A frequently heard concern about medication for the treatment of ADHD, particularly the stimulants, is the potential for abuse, both by the individual who has been prescribed the medication and by those who have unprescribed access (theft or sale of the medications to others). In fact, for individuals with ADHD, the opposite has been reported; the risk of abuse of other drugs is reduced when properly treated for ADHD.[33] Swedish researchers who studied almost 39,000 people with ADHD reported the following:[34]

1. There was no evidence of increased substance abuse.
2. There was evidence of decreased substance abuse four years after taking stimulant medications.
3. Longer duration of medication use was correlated with lower rates of abuse in both adults and adolescents with ADHD using stimulant medications.

These findings have been supported in other research.[35]

Nonetheless, these medications may fall into the hands of those for whom they have not been prescribed, and where the medications can be abused. This diversion of drugs from their intended users is of particular concern on college campuses, where as many as 1 in 20 students reported illicit use of ADHD stimulant medications.[36]

College students report several reasons why they used illicitly obtained stimulant medications, such as needing to stay awake and to focus on academic work and wanting to stay awake and be energetic for all-night social events. Other reasons for stimulant use among college students include the desire to be more social and outgoing, to lose weight, and to experience the energetic and powerful feeling it gives them.[37] Often these stimulant medications are combined with alcohol, marijuana, pain medications, or other drugs, making potential complications increase.[38] In one study it was reported that more than half of unprescribed ADHD medication users combine their stimulant use with alcohol, marijuana, or pain medication.[39]

If you suspect an adverse reaction to stimulant usage, either prescribed or not, follow local protocols for intervention, being sure to protect the airway if they are vomiting or have decreased mental status.

Cardiovascular events

Serious cardiovascular events, including sudden death, are reported as a rare but frightening side effect of ADHD medication. Most research does not support this concern, however. Some researchers believe a healthy person bias in these studies could be hiding the true cardiovascular risk from chronic use of stimulants.[40]

Habel et al. report that in their study of more than 150,000 ADHD medication users,[41] they found no evidence of increased risk of ECG changes, heart attack, or sudden cardiac death. In their review of several studies, Cortese et al.[42] did not find an increased risk of adverse cardiovascular events other than mild increases in heart rate and blood pressure for most people, and significant but sporadic tachycardia or hypertension in less than 15% of people taking ADHD medications. They recommend screening for preexisting cardiac conditions and periodic monitoring of heart rate and blood pressure, with ECGs only when clinically indicated.

Sinha et al.[43] suggest that adults with ADHD may be more at risk for adverse cardiovascular events due to an increased incidence of unhealthy lifestyles, including smoking, obesity, and substance use/abuse, along with the use of multiple medications to treat conditions comorbid with ADHD. They describe a case of one adult with ADHD with prescribed stimulant medication use who had a heart attack combined with new onset of atrial fibrillation. He subsequently was found to have no other drugs in his system that could explain a heart attack. His heart was seen to be healthy via an echo-cardiogram, and angiography showed no coronary artery disease. His final diagnosis was acute myocardial infarction with atrial fibrillation secondary to mixed amphetamine salts prescribed for his ADHD.

Most physicians consider the primary concerns associated with the cardiac health of adults with ADHD taking prescribed stimulants to be the potential for an increase in heart rate and blood pressure, along with the small increased risk for heart attack or stroke compared to adults not taking stimulants.[44]

An overdose of a stimulant medication can cause a very rapid heart rate, such as supraventricular tachycardia (SVT). The typical intervention, which is administration of adenosine, may cause refractory SVT. You can also consider the administration of a benzodiazepine, which may resolve the SVT.[45]

Depression

ADHD is associated with several comorbid conditions, including depression. The rate of depression is higher in people with ADHD (reported to be as high as 50%),[46] and the medications used to treat ADHD have often been considered as the source of the depression. A four-year study following almost 39,000 people with ADHD looking at the association of ADHD medications with depression found that instead of increasing the risk for depression, medication use was actually associated with a decreased risk for depression.[47] It is important to remember, however, that depression is independently associated with ADHD, and you may be called to support an individual with both disorders.

Suicidal ideation

Despite being listed as a serious potential side-effect for many medications, especially antidepressants, Cortese et al.[48] report that "there is little compelling evidence" that the rate of suicide in children being treated with ADHD medications is greater when compared to the general population. They speculate that the increased risk may be due in part to the comorbid disorders associated with ADHD or the ADHD itself, not necessarily the medication being used to treat the ADHD. All suicidal thoughts and behaviors, however, should be taken seriously, and you may be called to transport a patient having suicidal thoughts or who has attempted suicide. You should be prepared to treat injuries as needed and transport accordingly.

Implications for EMS

In the absence of other factors, the condition of ADHD is unlikely to precipitate an EMS response, but some of the related issues could result in the need for emergency care and transport. Treat the issues as they present, being sure to follow local protocols for treatment for substance overdose, including calling a poison control center for guidance.

Anxiety

Barbara, a 69-year-old woman, called 911 early one morning around 0700 complaining of chest pain and dizziness. The ALS chase vehicle arrives as the BLS ambulance is attempting their initial assessment. They state they have been unable to gather much information as the patient is agitated. Barbara is speaking rapidly, waving her arms around as she gestures, which causes the automatic blood pressure to time out. She describes her pain on onset as, "383 out of 10," with a reported time of onset at about 0600. Barbara is visibly anxious, stating she took two Ativan and Prozac prior to your arrival. She reports diagnoses of anxiety and OCD. Barbara has rapid, pressured speech, making assessment questions difficult. Her vitals are slightly elevated, with a heart rate of 116 and blood pressure of 146/83. When told that her 12-lead EKG shows nothing concerning, Barbara states she must be having heartburn and doesn't want to go to the hospital.

After some convincing, Barbara agrees to the transport. Throughout transport, she continues to talk rapidly, asking multiple questions about if she is dying, if her heart rhythm is normal, if she will be admitted, if you are being honest when telling her that her vitals are within normal limits, etc. Completing a full evaluation is difficult because every question you ask or vital sign you attempt to measure unleashes a new barrage of anxiety-driven questions (about why you are asking, what you think is wrong with her, if the doctor at the ED will be competent, and if the nurses will be friendly), making it impossible to obtain a complete history or ask follow-up questions. Upon arrival at the ED, she is so amped up with anxiety that the receiving nurse asks if she is drunk.

The DSM-5 identifies a variety of disorders that have characteristics of excessive fear and anxiety. *Fear* is defined as "the emotional response to real or perceived imminent threat," and *anxiety* is defined as the "anticipation of future threat."[49]

Anxiety Disorders That Might Precipitate an EMS Response

Panic disorder

Panic disorder may be diagnosed when the person has recurrent, unexpected panic attacks that are "abrupt surge[s] of intense fear or intense discomfort"[50] and include four or more physiological symptoms, such as palpitations, tachycardia, shaking, feelings of shortness of breath or choking, chest pain/discomfort, nausea, dizziness, numbness or tingling, feelings of detachment or unreality, and/or fears of losing control or death. Panic disorder has a prevalence of 2% to 3% in the United States, with a median age of onset around 20 to 24 years. It is rarely seen in pediatrics.

For a diagnosis, panic attacks must be *recurrent* (occur more than once) and *unexplained* (have no obvious cause or trigger). They can occur with varying degrees of frequency from daily to a few times a year. Sometimes people can have clusters of attacks, having them daily for several days, then none for months. A diagnosis of panic disorder carries a higher risk of suicide and suicidal ideation. Having the disorder leads to increased missed work or school, more emergency department and primary care visits, and a poorer quality of life.[51]

Panic disorder and subsequent panic attacks can be a frequent source of 911 calls as the symptoms can be very similar to respiratory distress or cardiac problems. As many as one-third of patients presenting to the emergency department with chest pain have panic disorder but may not have been diagnosed with panic disorder or may not reveal a mental health diagnosis for fear of being stigmatized or not being taken seriously.[52] They may also present with the physical symptoms of chest pain, palpitations, shortness of breath, sweating, shaking, and the like, but without the characteristic fear of death or losing control.[53] Consequently the patient may not recognize that they are having a panic attack.

There is a documented relationship between noncardiac chest pain and panic disorder, but rather than the chest pain being a symptom of the panic disorder, it is likely an independent condition that may be exacerbated by the anxiety.[54] It is important to conduct a thorough history and medical exam to rule out an underlying cause. It can be difficult even for emergency department physicians, however, to recognize the presenting symptoms as a panic attack.[55] Assuming that a patient's chest pain or other physical symptoms are related to or are worsened by their panic disorder, no matter how obvious you might think it is, can be potentially disastrous. Legitimate medical issues can cause feelings similar to a panic attack. This is a situation where EMS should assume a cardiac or respiratory etiology until proven otherwise.

Generalized anxiety disorder

Generalized anxiety disorder (*GAD*) may be experienced by individuals who are not able to control excessive anxiety and worry about events in their daily lives. For purposes of diagnosis, the worry must be accompanied by three of the following: restlessness, fatigue, difficulty concentrating, irritability, muscle tension, and/or sleep disturbances.[56] It is often accompanied by physical symptoms such as nausea, diarrhea, tachycardia, shortness of breath, headache, and dizziness.

The prevalence in the United States is just under 3% for adults and just under 1% for adolescents. The median age of onset is 30 years, but it can occur at any age.[57] GAD is estimated to have as high as 90% comorbidity with other psychiatric disorders such as depression and panic disorder.[58]

Generalized anxiety disorder can have associated physical symptoms that can be distressing or uncomfortable, including sleep disturbances, gastrointestinal problems, and headaches.[59] Additionally, research supports that people who are living with chronic illness are at increased risk for anxiety. These illnesses can make the anxiety worse and/or the anxiety can exacerbate the physical illness.[60] Afridi et al. found a correlation between irritable bowel disorder and GAD,[61] and Ahmed et al. found that people living with rheumatoid arthritis (RA) were often found to also have GAD.[62] For those individuals with both RA and GAD, the rheumatoid arthritis symptoms were more severe than for people with only RA.

Generalized anxiety disorder is not likely to precipitate an EMS call by itself. Even so, the excessive worry associated with the disorder, along with correlated physical illnesses, may mean that patients could call 911 for more minor issues that they fear could worsen. They may also experience more severe symptoms of their illness or associate more severity to symptoms than may be warranted.

When responding to a patient who is living with generalized anxiety disorder, it is important for you to acknowledge their concerns, take a thorough history, and conduct a complete assessment. Recognition that their concerns and fears are real to them is an important part of developing a relationship with your patient. You need to be cautious not to attribute symptoms as "just part of their anxiety" and potentially miss a serious problem.

Other Types of Anxiety Disorders

Selective mutism

Selective mutism is a failure to speak in social situations when there is an expectation of speaking, such as at school or during family events.[63] Children with selective mutism are able to speak, but they do not initiate or reciprocate in conversational opportunities with others. They will speak with immediate family members in their home but may not talk with extended family members or nonfamily members, such as teachers, clergy, or EMS providers. Children with selective mutism may also have delays in expressive language, social skills, and overall development.[64] Their receptive language (their understanding of what is said to them), however, is typically in the average to above-average range.[65] No clear, single cause of selective mutism has been found, but possible contributing factors include other anxiety disorders, genetics, environmental factors (limited social opportunities), and temperament.[66]

The American Speech-Language-Hearing Association notes that children with selective mutism may also have social anxiety and phobia.[67] They may exhibit the following:

- Separation anxiety, or refusal to separate from their parents
- Poor eye contact
- Running away or freezing in an uncomfortable or frightening situation
- Tantrums, especially if asked to speak
- Avoidance of public places

When encountering a patient with selective mutism, work with the patient's family members to obtain needed information. Other suggestions for interacting with children with selective mutism include the following:[68]

- Do not force the child to speak.
- Minimize eye contact. Sit or stand to the side of the child so you are not face to face with them.

- Allow for processing and thinking time.
- Encourage nonverbal communication attempts (head nodding, facial expressions, drawing, writing, etc.).
- Allow the child to choose the form of communication (writing, drawing, gesturing, etc.).
- Encourage whispering if the child is comfortable doing so.
- Allow parents/caregivers to stay with the child and encourage communication between parent and child.
- Stay calm and neutral in your responses and demeanor.

Agoraphobia

Agoraphobia is a significant fear or anxiety about being outside the home, in open spaces, in a crowd, in enclosed places where escape is difficult (e.g., elevator, crowded room), or using public transportation (fear of two or more of these situations is required for diagnosis).[69]

People with agoraphobia actively avoid situations that create fear or anxiety, and the feelings generated by the situation are out of proportion to the real dangers that may occur. They may be unable to leave the house or ride in a vehicle without intense fear. This can lead people to avoid or neglect needed preventative medical care and make it difficult to convince them to agree to transport to a hospital in a medical or traumatic emergency.

Additional Implications for EMS

- Keep your voice and body calm. Do not escalate an already anxious situation.
- Recognize that their anxiety is very real to them, even if you think their responses are unreasonable or overstated.
- Do not neglect to conduct a complete assessment, even if you think (or they say) it is an anxiety or panic attack. As noted previously, there are several potentially serious medical conditions that can mimic anxiety or panic.

Mood Disorders

You are dispatched for a 36-year-old woman, Olivia, who reports she is feeling suicidal. She has a history of being treated for chronic depression. A long-term relationship recently ended, deepening her depression and exacerbating her feelings of despair. Although she has not attempted suicide in the past, she is thinking about taking pills now because she "just can't take it anymore." She admits to drinking several glasses of wine before calling 911 for help. You conduct a thorough physical assessment, including blood sugar. All of her vital signs are within expected parameters. You help Olivia to the ambulance, secure her safely to the stretcher, and talk with her reassuringly as you transport her, without lights and sirens, to the emergency department for a psychiatric evaluation.

Mood disorders, such as depression and bipolar disorder, are some of the most common psychiatric disorders. According to a 2007 Harvard Medical School report, almost 10% of adults in the United States had a mood disorder, with rates being higher for women (11.6%) than men (7.7%).[70] Over 21% of adults in the United States have experienced a mood disorder at least once in their lives. Among adolescents aged 13 to 18, 14% were reported to have had a mood disorder, with the prevalence higher for females (18.3%) than males (10.5%).[71]

Depression

Depression is manifested by a variety of symptoms lasting at least two weeks, including the following:[72]

- Feelings of sadness, emptiness, or hopelessness
- Loss of interest or pleasure in activities
- Weight loss or weight gain
- Sleeping too much or not able to sleep
- Feeling restless or slow
- Lack of energy
- Feeling worthless
- Trouble concentrating or making decisions
- Thoughts of death or suicidal ideation

The depression must also have a significantly negative impact on work or social functioning. A person may exhibit depression-like symptoms after experiencing a significant loss, death of a loved one, or serious illness/injury, which can be part of the normal response to the experience.

Bipolar disorders

Bipolar disorders have also been called *manic-depressive disorders*. The DSM-5, or *Diagnostic and Statistical Manual of Mental Disorders*, fifth edition, describes several types of bipolar disorders, with bipolar I and bipolar II being the most familiar.[73] Bipolar disorders are characterized by periods of mania or "abnormally and persistently elevated, expansive, or irritable mood, and abnormally and persistently increased goal-directed activity or energy, lasting at least 1 week," coupled with periods of severe depression.[74] Bipolar disorder often begins to emerge in adolescence, with the first outward manifestation being a manic or hypomanic episode.[75]

The symptoms of depression associated with bipolar disorder are the same as seen in unipolar depression listed above.

Mania presents with a variety of signs and symptoms, including the following:[76]

- Inflated self-esteem
- Grandiosity
- Decreased need for sleep
- Excessive talking
- Racing thoughts
- Distractibility
- Increased goal-directed activity
- Psychomotor agitation
- Involvement in risky behaviors or activities that can have significant negative consequences

Mania also has a significantly negative impact on work or social functioning and may require hospitalization.

As previously mentioned, bipolar disorder types include *bipolar I* and *bipolar II*.

Bipolar I

Bipolar I is a disorder characterized by mania lasting at least one week, preceded and/or followed by a major depressive episode lasting at least two weeks.[77]

Bipolar II

In bipolar II disorder, the manic symptoms, while still present, are less severe, do not last as long as with bipolar I, do not significantly interfere with social or work functioning, and do not require hospitalization. This is called *hypomania.* The depressive manifestations are the same as with bipolar I.[78] The presence of a full manic episode rules out bipolar II.

Cyclothymia

People with *cyclothymia* have several periods with hypomanic symptoms that are not severe enough to meet the criteria for hypomania and periods of depressive symptoms that do not meet the criteria for depression. These symptoms must be present most of the time for at least two years in adults and one year in children and adolescents for diagnosis.[79]

Treatment for bipolar disorders

Standard therapeutic interventions for bipolar disorder in both adults and children include pharmacotherapy. Medications could include antipsychotics and mood stabilizers, with psychotherapy and ongoing monitoring of medication. Ongoing care and regular follow-up visits for managing the disorder are often infrequent, even when patients have readily available access to ongoing care.[80]

Complications associated with bipolar disorder

- *Cardiovascular disease.* Vascular disease, both cardiovascular and cerebrovascular, is the leading cause of death for people with bipolar disorder, even greater than death by suicide.[81] Other comorbid concerns associated with bipolar disorder include obesity, diabetes, hypertension, and hyperlipidemia, which are associated with the development of cardiovascular disease.[82] Some medications used to treat bipolar disorder cause weight gain, which is subsequently linked to cardiovascular disease. Smoking is also more common in people with bipolar disorder.[83]

- *Overdose.* People with mental health disorders are at greater risk for overdose, both deliberate and unintentional. In one study conducted by Buykx et al., patients reported inadequate mental health care as a contributing factor.[84] In addition, the act of overdosing, even when deliberate, did not correlate to an ultimate desire for death. Some were looking for a "temporary escape."[85]

- *Suicide.* People with bipolar disorder are at high risk for suicide, with a rate 10 to 30 times that of the general population.[86] Within the population of people with bipolar disorder in this study, women were nearly twice as likely to die by suicide and to have had previous attempts. Overdose (poisoning) was cited as the leading cause of suicide deaths.[87] Having a previous suicide attempt is a very strong predictor of a future attempt, especially in the first year after an earlier attempt.[88]

Implications for EMS

- You may be called for someone experiencing a new onset of mania, which can be manifested by agitation, irritation, or risky behavior. Be cautious of scene safety and personal safety.

- Be compassionate and nonjudgmental.

- Call poison control for guidance on medication overdoses and treat according to local protocols.

- If you suspect the patient may be planning to hurt themselves, do not leave them alone. You can consider asking them if they have thoughts of suicide or a plan to carry out the act of suicide. This is important information to give the emergency department so they provide the necessary support to ensure the patient remains safe once in their care.

- Be sure to do a thorough assessment and do not assume that a call for a behavioral problem does not have a medical component.

Obsessive-Compulsive Disorder

Alexandra is a 19-year-old college student with a diagnosis of obsessive-compulsive disorder. Her roommate called 911 when Alexandra appeared to be stuck in her compulsive routines of checking her belongings, ensuring the doors and windows were secured, and verifying that the appliances were turned off. Her routines were getting increasingly longer, she was skipping meals to complete her checking routines, and she was not sleeping well. When Alexandra's roommate was unable to gain her attention and break the frantic checking of the room, she called 911. Your arrival to the room stops her behaviors long enough for you to speak with her. You explain that her friends are concerned about her behavior and that she has not been eating or sleeping. Alexandra reveals to you that since she started attending college, she has run out of her medication and has been unable to refill her prescription because she has no transportation to a pharmacy. She agrees to go with you to the emergency department to get her medication refilled and to be evaluated.

Obsessive-compulsive disorder (*OCD*) is a chronic and common psychiatric or mental health disorder manifested by both obsessive and/or compulsive thoughts and behaviors. The DSM-5 defines *obsessions* as "recurrent and persistent thoughts, urges, or images that are experienced as intrusive and unwanted" and *compulsions* as "repetitive behaviors or mental acts that an individual feels driven to perform in response to an obsession or according to rules that must be applied rigidly."[89] Examples of possible obsessions and compulsions are listed in table 6–2. These lists are not exhaustive.

OCD is a common disorder, at slightly more than 1% of the population, with females being more at risk than males.[90] There is also increased comorbidity with autism spectrum disorders,[91] schizophrenia,[92] anxiety,[93] and depression.[94]

Table 6–2. A list of obsessions and compulsions

List of Obsessions and Compulsions	
Obsessions	**Compulsions**
• Worry about contamination and germs • Thoughts of losing control and harming self or others • Concerns about personal health • Intrusive violent thoughts • Thoughts about religion or morality • Thoughts of losing belongings • Need for strict order or symmetry • Intrusive sexual thoughts or fears of inappropriate sexual behavior • Worry that important tasks have been left undone (paying bills, keeping home clean, locking up home)	• Frequent hand washing or other grooming (teeth brushing, showering, etc.) • Frequent, excessive cleaning • Frequent checking of locks, appliances, welfare of others • Repetitive behaviors like tapping, counting items, activities (going in and out of doors or up and down stairs) often in multiples (the need to repeat words or activities three times, for example) • Rearranging or reordering items • Collecting things • Skin/nail picking or hair pulling

OCD can have a detrimental effect on the individual's quality of life and can worsen during times of stress. Living with OCD impacts an individual's social, occupational, cognitive, and family functioning.[95] OCD can lead to problems with social relationships and job functioning, but more concerning is the potential impact on cognitive functioning, resulting in memory impairment, poor decision-making skills, and poor inhibition. Family functioning can also be impacted, leading to marriage problems, financial concerns, and poor relationships within the family.[96]

Implications for EMS

- You may be called for patients experiencing a mental health crisis associated with their OCD. They may get "stuck" in their obsessive thoughts or in a compulsion (door checking or other repetitive behavior).[97]

- Acknowledge their behaviors and compulsions without judgment, ridicule, or amusement.
- Allow them to act on their need to perform the behaviors as long as you and they remain safe and there is no interference with patient care or transport. Not being able to act on the behaviors can increase anxiety.
- Engage them in conversation to help divert their thoughts from the obsession to something else.

Post-Traumatic Stress Disorder

Your tones drop for a 26-year-old male with a psychiatric emergency and possible overdose. After the scene has been secured by law enforcement, you locate your patient, Devon, on the third floor of a townhouse, sitting on the floor of the bathroom and refusing to move or speak. Family members tell you Devon recently returned from his second tour in Afghanistan after being injured with an improvised explosive device. They tell you they were having dinner on the outside deck when they heard a hunting rifle being shot in the distance. They said Devon went inside, and when he did not return to the meal, they found him shut up in the bathroom and refusing to come out. They were able to open the door and found him with an empty pill bottle. You check the bottle and see a prescription for 15-milligram oxycodone tablets. The prescription bottle, which was filled two days ago with 20 tablets, is empty. Devon's mental status is deteriorating. You place him on capnography to monitor his respiratory status, prepare to administer naloxone and provide ventilatory support if he experiences respiratory depression, and transport him to the hospital.

Post-traumatic stress disorder (PTSD) is a disorder with complex criteria for diagnosis as laid out in the DSM-5.[98] First the individual must have been exposed to death, serious injury, violence, and/or sexual violence, either through direct, personal experience by witnessing it as it was occurring, or from learning that a close family member or friend has experienced a significant trauma. This trauma experience can come from a single event such as a car accident or school shooting where someone was killed or seriously injured, or it can result from a pattern of ongoing exposure, such as domestic violence or child abuse.

In addition, the individual must have at least one of the following symptoms associated with the trauma:[99]

- Frequent and distressing memories of the trauma
- Distressing or frightening dreams about the event
- Flashbacks to the event
- Prolonged psychological distress when exposed to things that may remind them of the event (may be symbolic or representative rather than concrete)
- Physiological responses when exposed to things that may remind them of the event

They must also exhibit avoidance of memories and feelings of the traumatic event, as well as avoidance of reminders (people, places, activities, etc.) associated with the trauma.

Two or more of the following must also be present:[100]

- Irritable behavior and outbursts manifested as verbal or physical aggression
- Reckless behavior
- Self-destructive behavior
- Hypervigilance
- Exaggerated startle response
- Poor concentration
- Sleep disturbances

PTSD can be easy to overlook or misdiagnose as it is frequently comorbid with other mental health conditions such as depression and anxiety. Some of the manifestations of PTSD are physiological, such as rapid heart rate or breathing, dizziness, nausea, and/or abdominal pain, which can lead to the psychological symptoms not being addressed or considered. In some cases, the intrusive thoughts and images could be mistaken for hallucinations or psychosis.[101]

In addition to the psychological and physiological symptoms associated with PTSD, people with PTSD may also be at increased risk for cardiovascular disease, alcohol use disorder, schizophrenia, bipolar disorder, and self-harm behavior.

Cardiovascular disease

Both behavioral and biological factors are associated with PTSD and contribute to the development of cardiovascular disease.[102] Research conducted on returning war veterans shows that they are more likely to develop an alcohol use disorder and have a greater risk of beginning smoking or resuming smoking after a period of quitting. These may be attempts to self-medicate the symptoms of PTSD but can subsequently increase the risk of cardiovascular disease. Returning soldiers were also found to have higher rates of obesity and diabetes compared to the general population.

People with PTSD have twice the risk for developing hypertension, which in turn raises the risk for cardiovascular disease, according to research by Burg and Soufer.[103] An increase in heart rate, blood pressure, and autonomic dysregulation in response to stressful stimuli can lead to cardiac events.

More significantly, Burg and Soufer report that endothelium dysfunction is directly related to an increased risk of cardiovascular disease and adverse events.[104] The *endothelium* is described as a "single layer of cells that lines the lumen of all blood vessels, and serves as a bidirectional, biocompatible barrier that facilitates the passage of blood gases and a range of molecules to and from tissues so as to maintain vascular homeostasis."[105] Simply put, the endothelium is responsible for maintaining vascular tone. When the endothelium is not responding properly, it significantly increases the risk for cardiovascular disease. During times of emotional stress the endothelium can be dysfunctional, leading to vasoconstriction, potentially triggering cardiac events. This is significant for people with PTSD as they are experiencing increased levels of emotional dysregulation and stress.

Alcohol use disorder

PTSD is strongly comorbid with alcohol use disorder. People with PTSD may have two to three times greater risk of developing an alcohol use disorder when compared to the general population. People with PTSD are at a higher risk for any substance use disorder, but alcohol is the most commonly abused substance. This is particularly true for the veteran population, where reportedly 70% of veterans diagnosed with PTSD also had a substance use disorder, primarily using alcohol.[106]

The consequences of comorbid PTSD and alcohol use disorder include exacerbated of PTSD symptoms, suicidal ideation/attempts, poorer health overall, and the health risks associated independently with alcohol use disorders.[107]

Schizophrenia and bipolar disorder

A Danish study conducted on the relationship of PTSD to schizophrenia and bipolar disorder found that "the risk of developing schizophrenia, schizophrenia spectrum disorder, and bipolar affective disorder was more than 15-fold increased in the first year" after diagnosis of a traumatic stress disorder.[108]

Self-harm

People with PTSD are at greater risk for self-harm and suicide. The most common methods of self-harm are cutting, punching walls or objects, burning, hitting themselves, head banging, and skin/wound picking.[109]

Implications for EMS

- Be cautious about scene safety as individuals with PTSD are at risk for aggression.[110] Do not raise your voice to the individual or approach or touch them without letting them know what you intend to do. You do not want to exacerbate their response or frighten them.

- Do not minimize their experience or their response to the experience. Everyone responds to events differently. You may have been in a serious accident yourself, or you may be a combat veteran who has not experienced PTSD. That does not mean they are weak or your experience was not significant. It just means that each of you has responded differently.

- Do not threaten or give them ultimatums about transport to the hospital. Work with them until they can make a decision. Don't lie or trick them into making a decision.

- Remain calm so you do not escalate the situation.

- Give them space so they do not feel threatened or trapped.

- Ask them what they need from you so you can help them.

- If the person has overdosed on drugs or alcohol, be prepared to treat as appropriate with naloxone, airway management, and/or antidotes.

- Table 6–3 has suggestions for helping during a flashback to the traumatic event.
- Being a calm, understanding, nonjudgmental presence can go a long way in helping the individual through the crisis that precipitated the EMS response. Listen to them. Recognize that their feelings are very real and very powerful, and in that moment, they cannot control their behavior.

Table 6–3. Suggestions for helping during a flashback to the traumatic event

Suggestions for Helping during a Flashback to the Traumatic Event
• Remind them that it is a flashback and it is not actually happening again.
• Help them regain their grounding in the present by having them describe their current surroundings.
• Encourage them to take deep, slow breaths to prevent hyperventilating. Count their breaths with them and talk them through slow, regular breaths.
• Avoid sudden movements or anything that might startle them.
• Do not touch them without their permission.

Source: Adapted from Melinda Smith and Lawrence Robinson, "Helping Someone with PTSD," HelpGuide, January 2018, retrieved April 21, 2018, https://www.helpguide.org/articles/ptsd-trauma/helping-someone-with-ptsd.htm.

Schizophrenia

You are called to a local group home for people with mental health disorders. The dispatch reason is nonspecific, stating you are responding for a 26-year-old male with a psychiatric emergency. Law enforcement is en route, and you proceed in after they secure the scene. Your patient, Kyle, is calm and alert. He is oriented to self, place, and time. When you ask how you can help him today, Kyle replies that he is being pursued by zombies and fears for his safety. After getting his permission, you conduct a physical exam, including blood sugar, and find nothing out of the ordinary. After reassuring Kyle that you will take him to the hospital where he will be safe and empathizing that what he is experiencing must be frightening, you help him to the ambulance for a routine transport to the closest emergency department.

Schizophrenia is a severe mental health disorder that can contribute to the need for EMS intervention and subsequent transport to the emergency department. In addition to the psychiatric symptoms, people with schizophrenia are at increased risk for a variety of physical health complications secondary to their mental health disorder.

The DSM-5 describes *schizophrenia* as a psychotic disorder with the following five components:[111]

- *Delusions*. Delusions are beliefs that do not change, even when there is evidence that they are not accurate. Delusions can take many forms, including *persecutory* (believing that other people or groups are going to harm you), *referential* (believing that other people's behaviors or words are directed at you), grandiose (believing that you have exceptional skills or are wealthy or famous), *erotomanic* (believing that someone is in love with you when they are not), *nihilistic* (believing that a catastrophe will happen), and *somatic* (intense focus on your health and well-being).

- *Hallucinations*. Hallucinations are experiences that feel real but are not actually happening. They can occur with all the senses, but auditory hallucinations are the most common.

- *Disorganized thinking*. Disorganized thinking is a thought disorder that is observed through a person's speech. When thoughts are disorganized, the person may switch quickly between topics, answer questions with off-topic or unrelated responses, and/or their speech may be incomprehensible or incoherent.

- *Disorganized or abnormal motor behavior*. This behavior can range from agitation, silliness, and excessive movement to *catatonia* (diminished reactions to environmental stimuli), odd posturing, no speech or physical responses, stereotypical movements, or echolalia.

- *Negative symptoms*. These symptoms are a loss of function and can include a reduction in emotional expression (facial expressions, tone of voice, gestures), a decrease in purposeful activities, reduced speech output, an inability to experience pleasure, and a lack of interest in social interactions.

Emergency department visits for this disorder are high, and men with schizophrenia have more than twice as many visits as women with schizophrenia. Half of these emergency department visits lead to either hospital admission or psychiatric hospital admission.[112]

While the psychiatric manifestations of schizophrenia can lead to emergency transport to the hospital to address these symptoms, there are many comorbid conditions that may also necessitate emergency care. These should not be dismissed as part of the person's mental health symptoms, and neither should they be assumed to be irrelevant or less severe because the person has a significant and serious mental health disorder.

The two most common comorbid conditions associated with schizophrenia are type II diabetes and depression.[113] Compared to the general population, depression is reported to be up to six times more common in people with schizophrenia. Type II diabetes is twice as prevalent in people with schizophrenia.

Diabetes

The link between diabetes and schizophrenia is multifaceted and can be related to psychiatric medication usage and lifestyle habits. Antipsychotic medications can have adverse pancreatic and metabolic effects. These effects can lead to weight gain and hyperglycemia, which are associated with the development of type II diabetes. There are also psychosocial contributions as many people with schizophrenia are living in situations that do not allow for healthy eating, exercise, and/or self-care, which can contribute to the development and worsening of type II diabetes.[114]

People with schizophrenia and diabetes are at increased risk for hospitalization for hypoglycemia, hyperglycemia, and infection associated with diabetes. The mortality rate is almost twice as high for diabetics with schizophrenia compared to people with only type II diabetes.[115]

While it could be assumed that diabetic complications in people with schizophrenia could be related to limited access to medical appointments and/or challenges with financing diabetes management (diabetes is an expensive disease to manage), this may be only part of the cause. In a study conducted in Canada, where health care is publicly funded and patients had good access to physicians, the authors found that people with diabetes and schizophrenia still had an increase in complications and poor outcomes.[116] They attributed these poor outcomes to patient factors, such as not being able to manage their diabetes well due to their mental illness, but also to physician factors, which included not feeling well-equipped to manage both the diabetes and the schizophrenia, time constraints, and stigma surrounding the mental health diagnosis.

Respiratory disease

Respiratory complications such as asthma and COPD are more prevalent in people with schizophrenia and can be associated with smoking (90% of people with schizophrenia are reported to smoke tobacco). Additionally, there is an association between nicotine addiction and depression. Attempts to stop smoking during a depressive event can prolong the depression.[117]

Respiratory infections such as pneumonia and bronchitis can be particularly dangerous for elderly patients with schizophrenia.[118]

Many other physical illnesses are found be at higher rates in people with schizophrenia, and comorbidities can contribute to the worsening of other illnesses.

Gastrointestinal problems

Gastrointestinal issues associated with schizophrenia have been documented for a long time.[119] These issues can be attributed to bowel motility issues associated with the use of antipsychotic medications and include constipation and bowel obstruction, as well as medication side effects such as nausea, vomiting, and pain.

Correlation between schizophrenia and chronic inflammatory gastrointestinal conditions such as irritable bowel syndrome, inflammatory bowel disease, Crohn's disease, and celiac disease have been reported.[120] Postmortem studies on patients with schizophrenia report very high rates of gastritis, enteritis, and colitis.

Eye abnormalities

Vision problems commonly occur in people with schizophrenia. These include not only the visual hallucinations that are part of the clinical diagnosis criteria, but also structural and functional problems of the eye that are reported to be not only comorbid with schizophrenia but may also be part of the disease process.[121]

- *Nystagmus* is a motor disorder in which the eyes move rapidly and uncontrollably horizontally, vertically, or in a circular pattern, which can have a negative impact on visual acuity, depth perception, and balance.[122] Nystagmus has been reported in 50% to 85% of people with schizophrenia, compared to 8% of the general population.[123]

- *Strabismus* (crossed eyes) is a misalignment of the muscles of the eyes, causing the eyes to turn in, turn out, or turn up. It can cause double vision and poor depth perception. Strabismus has a prevalence of 1% to 5% in the general population and as high as 13% in patients with schizophrenia.[124]

- *Poor visual acuity* can be attributed to medication side effects.[125]

Schizophrenia and intellectual disability

People with an intellectual disability have a significantly increased rate of schizophrenia (see chapter 3).[126] The schizophrenia associated with intellectual disability tends to have more negative symptoms (flat affect, limited speech, low energy, and social withdrawal) than those who have schizophrenia without intellectual disability.

Implications for EMS

- Be sure to check blood sugar in patients with schizophrenia. Do not assume an altered mental status is a manifestation of schizophrenia until you have ruled out hypoglycemia or hyperglycemia.

- Patients who are compliant with their antipsychotic medications and are experiencing severe abdominal pain may have a bowel obstruction.

- Do not argue with patients about their hallucinations or delusions and tell them they do not exist or they are wrong. Neither should you lie and say that you also see, hear, or believe them. You can acknowledge that you understand what they are experiencing is real to them and reassure them that you are there to support them and keep them safe.

- Do not assume that the reason for the 911 call is solely psychiatric. It is easy to get tunnel vision and assume that the patient just needs transport for a psychiatric evaluation or admission. Do not neglect to conduct a thorough assessment to rule out medical issues that can and should be treated.

Notes

1. US Dept. of Health and Human Services, National Institutes of Health, National Institute of Mental Health, "Mental Illness," November 2017, retrieved February 3, 2018, https://www.nimh.nih.gov/health/statistics/mental-illness.shtml.

2. Craig W. Colton and Ronald W. Manderscheid, "Congruencies in Increased Mortality Rates, Years of Potential Life Lost, and Causes of Death among Public Mental Health Clients in Eight States," *Preventing Chronic Disease* 3, no. 2 (2006): 1–14, https://www.ncbi.nlm.nih.gov/pmc/articles/PMC1563985/pdf/PCD32A42.pdf; and US Department of Housing and Urban Development, Office of Community Planning and Development, *The 2010 Annual Homeless Assessment Report* (Washington, DC: US Department of Housing and Urban Development, 2010): 1–207.

3. Ingrid Waldron, "Communicating with a Loved One Who Has a Mental Illness," National Alliance on Mental Illness, NAMI Main Line PA, June 2014, retrieved February 3, 2018, https://namipamainline.org/communicating-with-a-loved-one-who-has-a-mental-illness/; and David F. Swink, "Communicating with People with Mental Illness: The Public's Guide," October 19, 2010, retrieved February 3, 2018, https://www.psychologytoday.com/blog/threat-management/201010/communicating-people-mental-illness-the-publics-guide.

4. Patricia Hentz, "Separating Anxiety from Physical Illness," *Clinical Advisor* 11, no. 3 (2008), http://www.clinicaladvisor.com/features/separating-anxiety-from-physical-illness/article/117767/.

5. Robert J. Hedaya, *Understanding Biological Psychiatry* (New York: W.W. Norton, 1996).

6. Hedaya, *Understanding Biological Psychiatry*.

7. N. Gregg et al., "Neurobehavioural Changes in Patients Following Brain Tumour: Patients and Relatives Perspective," *Supportive Care in Cancer* 22, no. 11 (2014): 2,965–2,972, https://doi.org/10.1007/s00520-014-2291-3; and Subramoniam Madhusoodanan et al, "Brain Tumor and Psychiatric Manifestations: A Case Report and Brief Review," *Annals of Clinical Psychiatry* 16, no. 2 (2004): 111–113, https://doi.org/10.1080/10401230490453770.

8. William Breitbart et al., "Depression, Cytokines, and Pancreatic Cancer," *Psycho-Oncology* 23, no. 3 (2013): 339–345, https://doi.org/10.1002/pon.3422.

9. J. Edge and E. Panieri, "Phaeochromocytoma—A Classic (But Easily Forgotten) Cause of Anxiety," *African Journal of Psychiatry* 14, no. 2 (2011): 154–156.

10. A. Talaei et al., "TSH Cut Off Point Based on Depression in Hypothyroid Patients," *BMC Psychiatry* 17, no. 327 (2017): 1–5, https://doi.org/10.1186/s12888-017-1478-9.

11. Karolina Jabłkowska et al., "Working Memory and Executive Functions in Hyperthyroid Patients with Graves' Disease," *Archives of Psychiatry and Psychotherapy* 1 (2009): 69–75; Murat Emul et al., "Thyrotoxic Psychosis in an Elderly Woman and Haloperidol Use: A Case Report," *Psychogeriatrics* 13, no. 1 (2013): 49–51, https://doi.org/10.1111/j.1479-8301.2012.00404.x; and Guru S. Gowda et al., "Psychosis Following Carbimazole-Induced Acute Alteration of Hyperthyroid Status," *Indian Journal of Psychological Medicine* 39, no. 4 (2017): 516–518, https://doi.org/10.4103/0253-7176.211753.

12. Alicia Santos et al., "Depression and Anxiety Scores Are Associated with Amygdala Volume in Cushing's Syndrome: Preliminary Study," *BioMed Research International* 2017, (2017): 1–7, https://doi.org/10.1155/2017/2061935; and C. Dimopoulou et al., "Increased Prevalence of Anxiety-Associated Personality Traits in Patients with Cushing's Disease: A Cross-Sectional Study," *Neuroendocrinology* 97, no. 2 (2013): 139–145, https://doi.org/10.1159/000338408.

13. US Dept. of Health and Human Services, National Institutes of Health, National Institute of Diabetes and Digestive and Kidney Diseases, "Adrenal Insufficiency and Addison's Disease," May 1, 2014, retrieved February 3, 2018, https://www.niddk.nih.gov/health-information/endocrine-diseases/adrenal-insufficiency-addisons-disease.

14. US Dept. of Health and Human Services, National Institutes of Health, National Institute of Diabetes and Digestive and Kidney Diseases, "Low Blood Glucose (Hypoglycemia)," August 1, 2016, retrieved February 3, 2018, https://www.niddk.nih.gov/health-information/diabetes/overview/preventing-problems/low-blood-glucose-hypoglycemia.

15. Gaurav Agarwal and Satish K. Singh, "Arrhythmias in Type 2 Diabetes Mellitus," *Indian Journal of Endocrinology and Metabolism* 21, no. 5 (2017): 715–718, https://doi.org/10.4103/ijem.ijem_448_16.

16. Lauren Vogel, "Growing Consensus on Link between Strep and Obsessive–Compulsive Disorder," *Canadian Medical Association Journal* 190, no. 3 (2018): E86–E87, https://doi.org/10.1503/cmaj.109-5545.

17. Emanuel Schattner et al., "Depression in Systemic Lupus Erythematosus: The Key Role of Illness Intrusiveness and Concealment of Symptoms," Psychiatry: Interpersonal and Biological Processes 73, no. 4 (2010): 329–340, https://doi.org/10.1521/psyc.2010.73.4.329; and M. A. Coín et al., "The Role of Antiphospholipid Autoantibodies in the Cognitive Deficits of Patients with Systemic Lupus Erythematosus," Lupus 24, no. 8 (2015): 875–879, https://doi.org/10.1177/0961203315572717.

18. Theresa A. Rowe and Manisha Juthani-Mehta, "Urinary Tract Infection in Older Adults," *Aging Health* 9, no. 5 (2013): 519–528, https://doi.org/10.2217/ahe.13.38.

19. N. Berry, R. Sagar, and B. M. Tripathi, "Catatonia and Other Psychiatric Symptoms with Vitamin B12 Deficiency," *Acta Psychiatrica Scandinavica* 108, no. 2 (2003): 156–159, https://doi.org/10.1034/j.1600-0447.2003.00089.x; C. Blundo, D. Marin, and M. Ricci, "Vitamin B12 Deficiency Associated with Symptoms of Frontotemporal Dementia," *Neurological Sciences* 32, no. 1 (2010): 101–105, https://doi.org/10.1007/s10072-010-0419-x; and C. Marcel, *Vitamin B12 Deficiency* (Glendale, CA: Cinahl Information Systems, 2017).

20. S. Dixon and C. Marcel, *Thiamin* (Glendale, CA: Cinahl Information Systems, 2017).

21. A. Spinneker et al., "Vitamin B6 Status, Deficiency, and Its Consequences—An Overview," *Nutricion Hospitalaria* 22, no. 1 (2007): 7–24; and C. Marcel, *Vitamin B6 Deficiency* (Glendale, CA: Cinahl Information Systems, 2017).

22. Jonathan M. Silver, Thomas W. McAllister, and Stuart C. Yudofsky, eds., *Textbook of Traumatic Brain Injury* (Washington, DC: American Psychiatric Publishing, 2005); and Suman Ahmed et al., "Traumatic Brain Injury and Neuropsychiatric Complications," *Indian Journal of Psychological Medicine* 39, no. 2 (2017): 114–121, https://doi.org/10.4103/0253-7176.203129.

23. Lucia Ricciardi et al., "Facial Emotion Recognition and Expression in Parkinson's Disease: An Emotional Mirror Mechanism?" *PLoS ONE* 12, no. 1 (2017): 1–16, https://doi.org/10.1371/journal.pone.0169110.

24. Suman Ahmed, Baptiste Leurent, and Elizabeth L. Sampson, "Risk Factors for Incident Delirium among Older People in Acute Hospital Medical Units: A Systematic Review and Meta-Analysis," *Age and Ageing* 43, no. 3 (2014): 326–333, https://doi.org/10.1093/ageing/afu022; Osman Özdemir et al., "Is There Any Relationship between Sodium and Depression?" Journal of Mood Disorders 4, no. 4 (2014): 163–166, https://doi.org/10.5455/jmood.20140609102738; and Sagarika Mukherjee et al., "Acute Psychological Stress-Induced Water Intoxication," *International Journal of Psychiatry in Clinical Practice* 9, no. 2 (2005): 142–144, https://doi.org/10.1080/13651500510028986.

25. American Psychiatric Association, *Diagnostic and Statistical Manual of Mental Disorders*, 5th ed. (Washington, DC: American Psychiatric Association, 2013).

26. APA, *Diagnostic and Statistical Manual of Mental Disorders*.

27. APA, *Diagnostic and Statistical Manual of Mental Disorders*.

28. APA, *Diagnostic and Statistical Manual of Mental Disorders*.

29. Francine Conway, Maria Oster, and Kate Szymanski, "ADHD and Complex Trauma: A Descriptive Study of Hospitalized Children in an Urban Psychiatric Hospital," *Journal of Infant, Child, and Adolescent Psychotherapy* 10, no. 1 (2011): 60–72, https://doi.org/10.1080/15289168.2011.575707.

30. Sean Lynch et al., "Toward Effective Utilization of the Pediatric Emergency Department: The Case of ADHD," *Social Work in Public Health* 31, no. 1 (2016): 9–18, https://doi.org/10.1080/19371918.2015.1087909.

31. Lynch et al., "Toward Effective Utilization of the Pediatric Emergency Department."

32. Lynch et al., "Toward Effective Utilization of the Pediatric Emergency Department," 15.

33. Scott H. Kollins, "Abuse Liability of Medications Used to Treat Attention-Deficit/Hyperactivity Disorder (ADHD)," *American Journal on Addictions* 16, no. S1 (2007): 35–44, https://doi.org/10.1080/10550490601082775.

34. Zheng Chang et al., "Stimulant ADHD Medication and Risk for Substance Abuse," *Journal of Child Psychology and Psychiatry* 55, no. 8 (2014): 878–885, https://doi.org/10.1111/jcpp.12164.

35. Patrick D. Quinn et al., "ADHD Medication and Substance-Related Problems," *American Journal of Psychiatry* 174, no. 9 (2017): 877–885, https://doi.org/10.1176/appi.ajp.2017.16060686; and Sean E. McCabe et al., "Age of Onset, Duration, and Type of Medication Therapy for Attention-Deficit/

Hyperactivity Disorder and Substance Use during Adolescence: A Multi-Cohort National Study," *Journal of the American Academy of Child & Adolescent Psychiatry* 55, no. 6 (2016): 479–486, https://doi.org/10.1016/j.jaac.2016.03.011.

36. Kollins, "Abuse Liability of Medications Used to Treat ADHD."

37. Alan D. DeSantis, Elizabeth M. Webb, and Seth M. Noar, "Illicit Use of ADHD Medications on a College Campus: A Multimethodological Approach," *Journal of American College Health* 57, no. 3 (2008): 315–324, https://doi.org/10.3200/jach.57.3.315-324.

38. L. Chen et al., "Patterns of Concurrent Substance Use among Adolescent Nonmedical ADHD Stimulant Users," *Addictive Behaviors* 49 (2015): 1–6, https://doi:10.1016/j.addbeh.2015.05.007.

39. Chen et al., "Patterns of Concurrent Substance Use."

40. Philip Shaw, "ADHD Medications and Cardiovascular Risk," *Journal of the American Medical Association* 306, no. 24 (2011): 2,723–2,724, https://doi.org/10.1001/jama.2011.1866.

41. Laurel A. Habel et al., "ADHD Medications and Risk of Serious Cardiovascular Events in Young and Middle-Aged Adults," *Journal of the American Medical Association* 306, no. 24 (2011): 2,673–2,683, https://doi.org/10.1001/jama.2011.1830.

42. Samuele Cortese et al., "Practitioner Review: Current Best Practice in the Management of Adverse Events during Treatment with ADHD Medications in Children and Adolescents," *Journal of Child Psychology and Psychiatry* 54, no. 3 (2013): 227–246, https://doi.org/10.1111/jcpp.12036.

43. A. Sinha et al., "Adult ADHD Medications and Their Cardiovascular Implications," *Case Reports in Cardiology* 2016: 1–6, https://doi.org/10.1155/2016/2343691.

44. Sinha et al., "Adult ADHD Medications and Their Cardiovascular Implications"; and Jan Sieluk et al., "ADHD Medications and Cardiovascular Adverse Events in Children and Adolescents: Cross-National Comparison of Risk Communication in Drug Labeling," *Pharmacoepidemiology and Drug Safety* 26, no. 3 (2017): 274–284, https://doi.org/10.1002/pds.4164.

45. Maryland Institute for Emergency Medical Services Systems, *Maryland Medical Protocols for Emergency Medical Services Providers* (Baltimore, MD: Maryland Institute for Emergency Medical Services Systems, 2018), 1–494.

46. Zheng Chang et al., "Medication for Attention-Deficit/Hyperactivity Disorder and Risk for Depression: A Nationwide Longitudinal Cohort Study," *Biological Psychiatry* 80, no. 12 (2016): 916–922, https://doi.org/10.1016/j.biopsych.2016.02.018.

47. Chang et al., "Medication for ADHD and Risk for Depression."

48. Samuele Cortese et al., "Practitioner Review: Current Best Practice," 238.

49. American Psychiatric Association, *Diagnostic and Statistical Manual of Mental Disorders*, 5th ed. (Washington, DC: APA, 2013), 189.

50. APA, *Diagnostic and Statistical Manual of Mental Disorders*, 208.

51. APA, *Diagnostic and Statistical Manual of Mental Disorders*.

52. Geneviève Belleville, Guillaume Foldes-Busque, and André Marchand, "Characteristics of Panic Disorder Patients Consulting an Emergency Department with Noncardiac Pain," *Primary Psychiatry* 17, no. 3 (2010): 35–42.

53. Belleville et al., "Characteristics of Panic Disorder Patients"; and Kyle W. Harvison, Janet Woodruff-Borden, and Sarah E. Jeffery, "Mismanagement of Panic Disorder in Emergency Departments: Contributors, Costs, and Implications for Integrated Models of Care," *Journal of Clinical Psychology in Medical Settings* 11, no. 3 (2004): 217–232, https://doi.org/10.1023/b:jocs.0000037616.60987.89.

54. Guillaume Foldes-Busque et al., "Factors Associated with Pain Level in Non-Cardiac Chest Pain Patients with Comorbid Panic Disorder," *BioPsychoSocial Medicine* 10, no. 1 (2016): 1–8, https://doi.org/10.1186/s13030-016-0081-5.

55. Harvison et al., "Mismanagement of Panic Disorder in Emergency Departments."

56. APA, *Diagnostic and Statistical Manual of Mental Disorders*.

57. APA, *Diagnostic and Statistical Manual of Mental Disorders*.

58. Zeynep E. Bal et al., "Temperament and Character Dimensions of Personality in Patients with Generalized Anxiety Disorder," *Journal of Mood Disorders* 7, no. 1 (2017): 10–19, https://doi.org/10.5455/jmood.20170214015231.

59. Zhen-Ni Guo et al., "Characteristics of Cardio-Cerebrovascular Modulation in Patients with Generalized Anxiety Disorder: An Observational Study," *BMC Psychiatry* 17, no. 1 (2017): 1–7, https://doi.org/10.1186/s12888-017-1428-6.

60. Louise Pelletier et al., "The Burden of Generalized Anxiety Disorder in Canada," *Health Promotion and Chronic Disease Prevention in Canada* 37, no. 2 (2017): 54–62, https://doi.org/10.24095/hpcdp.37.2.04.

61. H. Afridi et al., "Is There a Relationship between Irritable Bowel Syndrome and Generalized Anxiety Disorder?" *Journal of Postgraduate Medical Institute* 31, no. 3 (2017): 271–275.

62. Asmaa B. Ahmed, Abdulah M. A. Radwan, and Hamid M. Baddary, "Prevalence of Generalized Anxiety Disorder in Patients with Rheumatoid Arthritis and Its Relationship with Disease Activity," *Egyptian Journal of Hospital Medicine* 65 (2016): 652–661, https://doi.org/10.12816/0033778.

63. APA, *Diagnostic and Statistical Manual of Mental Disorders*.

64. Peter Muris and Thomas H. Ollendick, "Children Who Are Anxious in Silence: A Review on Selective Mutism, the New Anxiety Disorder in DSM-5," *Clinical Child and Family Psychology Review* 18, no. 2 (2015): 151–169, https://doi.org/10.1007/s10567-015-0181-y.

65. American Speech-Language-Hearing Association, "Selective Mutism," retrieved April 3, 2018, https://www.asha.org/Practice-Portal/Clinical-Topics/Selective-Mutism/.

66. ASHA, "Selective Mutism."

67. ASHA, "Selective Mutism."

68. Shu-Lan Hung, Michael S. Spencer, and Rani Dronamraju, "Selective Mutism: Practice and Intervention Strategies for Children," *Children & Schools* 34, no. 4 (2012): 222–230, https://doi.org/10.1093/cs/cds006; and ASHA, "Selective Mutism."

69. APA, *Diagnostic and Statistical Manual of Mental Disorders*.

70. Harvard Medical School, "Data Table 1: Lifetime Prevalence DSM-IV/WMH-CIDI Disorders by Sex and Cohort," *National Comorbidity Survey*, 2007, retrieved May 25, 2018 from https://www.hcp.med.harvard.edu/ncs/index.php; and Harvard Medical School, "Data Table 2: 12-Month Prevalence DSM-IV/WMH-CIDI Disorders by Sex and Cohort," *National Comorbidity Survey*, 2007, retrieved May 25, 2018 from https://www.hcp.med.harvard.edu/ncs/index.php.

71. Kathleen R. Merikangas et al., "Lifetime Prevalence of Mental Disorders in U.S. Adolescents: Results from the National Comorbidity Survey Replication--Adolescent Supplement (NCS-A)," *Journal of the American Academy of Child and Adolescent Psychiatry* 49, no. 10 (2010): 980–989, https://doi.org/10.1016/j.jaac.2010.05.017.

72. APA, *Diagnostic and Statistical Manual of Mental Disorders*.

73. APA, *Diagnostic and Statistical Manual of Mental Disorders*.

74. APA, *Diagnostic and Statistical Manual of Mental Disorders*, 124.

75. Daniel Dietch, "Recognising Bipolar Disorders in Primary Care," *Psychiatria Danubina* 27, supp. 1 (2015): S188–194.

76. APA, *Diagnostic and Statistical Manual of Mental Disorders*.

77. APA, *Diagnostic and Statistical Manual of Mental Disorders*.

78. APA, *Diagnostic and Statistical Manual of Mental Disorders*.

79. APA, *Diagnostic and Statistical Manual of Mental Disorders*.

80. Jennifer L. Vande Voort et al., "Treatments and Services Provided to Children Diagnosed with Bipolar Disorder," *Child Psychiatry & Human Development* 47, no. 3 (2016): 494–502, https://doi.org/10.1007/s10578-015-0582-7.

81. Miriam Weiner, Lois Warren, and Jess G. Fiedorowicz, "Cardiovascular Morbidity and Mortality in Bipolar Disorder," *Annals of Clinical Psychiatry* 23, no. 1 (2011): 40–47.

82. Weiner, Warren, and Fiedorowicz, "Cardiovascular Morbidity and Mortality in Bipolar Disorder."

83. Weiner, Warren, and Fiedorowicz, "Cardiovascular Morbidity and Mortality in Bipolar Disorder."

84. Penny Buykx et al., "Patients Who Attend the Emergency Department Following Medication Overdose: Self-Reported Mental Health History and Intended Outcomes of Overdose." *International Journal of Mental Health and Addiction* 10, no. 4 (2012): 501–511, https://doi.org/10.1007/s11469-011-9338-1.

85. Buykx et al., "Patients Who Attend the Emergency Department Following Medication Overdose," 509.

86. Ayal Schaffer et al., "Suicide in Bipolar Disorder: Characteristics and Subgroups," *Bipolar Disorders* 16, no. 7 (2014): 732–740, https://doi.org/10.1111/bdi.12219.

87. Schaffer et al., "Suicide in Bipolar Disorder."

88. M. H. Allen et al., "Screening for Suicidal Ideation and Attempts among Emergency Department Medical Patients: Instrument and Results from the Psychiatric Emergency Research Collaboration," *Suicide and Life-Threatening Behavior* 43, no. 3 (2013): 313–323, https://doi.org/10.1111/sltb.12018.

89. APA, *Diagnostic and Statistical Manual of Mental Disorders*, 235.

90. APA, *Diagnostic and Statistical Manual of Mental Disorders*.

91. Sandra M. Meier et al., "Obsessive-Compulsive Disorder and Autism Spectrum Disorders: Longitudinal and Offspring Risk," *PLoS ONE* 10, no. 11 (2015): 1–12, https://doi.org/10.1371/journal.pone.0141703.

92. Sandra M. Meier et al., "Obsessive-Compulsive Disorder as a Risk Factor for Schizophrenia," *JAMA Psychiatry* 71, no. 11 (2014): 1,215–1,221, https://doi.org/10.1001/jamapsychiatry.2014.1011.

93. I. Paul et al., "Co-Morbidity of Obsessive-Compulsive Disorder and Other Anxiety Disorders with Child and Adolescent Mood Disorders," *East Asian Archives of Psychiatry* 25 (2015): 58–63.

94. Paul et al., "Co-Morbidity of Obsessive-Compulsive Disorder and Other Anxiety Disorders with Child and Adolescent Mood Disorders."

95. Puspita Sahoo, Rati Ranjan Sethy, and Daya Ram, "Functional Impairment and Quality of Life in Patients with Obsessive Compulsive Disorder," *Indian Journal of Psychological Medicine* 39, no. 6 (2017): 760–765, https://doi.org/10.4103/ijpsym.ijpsym_53_17.

96. Sahoo et al., "Functional Impairment and Quality of Life in Patients with OCD."

97. Kelley Madick, "Care of the Patient with Obsessive-Compulsive Disorder," February 17, 2016, retrieved May 5, 2018, https://ceufast.com/course/obsessive-compulsive-disorder-ocd-for-the-cna.

98. APA, *Diagnostic and Statistical Manual of Mental Disorders*.

99. APA, *Diagnostic and Statistical Manual of Mental Disorders*.

100. APA, Diagnostic and Statistical Manual of Mental Disorders.

101. Ruth V. Reed, Mina Fazel, and Lorna Goldring, "Post-Traumatic Stress Disorder," *British Medical Journal* 344, no. 7,870 (2012): 44–45, https://doi.org/10.1136/bmj.e3790.

102. Matthew M. Burg and Robert Soufer, "Post-Traumatic Stress Disorder and Cardiovascular Disease," *Current Cardiology Reports* 18, no. 94 (2016): 1–7, https://doi.org/10.1007/s11886-016-0770-5.

103. Burg and Soufer, "Post-Traumatic Stress Disorder and Cardiovascular Disease."

104. Burg and Soufer, "Post-Traumatic Stress Disorder and Cardiovascular Disease."

105. Burg and Soufer, "Post-Traumatic Stress Disorder and Cardiovascular Disease," 3.

106. N. W. Gilpin and J. L. Weiner, "Neurobiology of Comorbid Post-Traumatic Stress Disorder and Alcohol-Use Disorder," *Genes, Brain and Behavior* 16, no. 1 (2017): 15–43, https://doi.org/10.1111/gbb.12349.

107. Gilpin and Weiner, "Neurobiology of Comorbid Post-Traumatic Stress Disorder and Alcohol-Use Disorder."

108. Niels Okkels et al., "Traumatic Stress Disorders and Risk of Subsequent Schizophrenia Spectrum Disorder of Bipolar Disorder: A Nationwide Cohort Study," *Schizophrenia Bulletin* 43, no. 1 (2017): 182, https://doi.org/10.1093/schbul/sbw082.

109. Kevin F. W. Dyer et al., "Anger, Aggression, and Self-Harm in PTSD and Complex PTSD," *Journal of Clinical Psychology* 65, no. 10 (2009): 1,099–1,114, https://doi.org/10.1002/jclp.20619.

110. Dyer et al., "Anger, Aggression, and Self-Harm in PTSD and Complex PTSD."

111. APA, *Diagnostic and Statistical Manual of Mental Disorders*.

112. Michael L. Albert and Linda McCaig, *Emergency Department Visits Related to Schizophrenia among Adults Aged 18–64: United States, 2009–2011*, Data Brief No. 215 (Hyattsville, MD: National Center for Health Statistics, 2015).

113. D. Schoepf et al., "Physical Comorbidity and Its Relevance on Mortality in Schizophrenia: A Naturalistic 12-Year Follow-Up in General Hospital Admissions," *European Archives of Psychiatry and Clinical Neuroscience* 264, no. 1 (2014): 3–28, https://doi.org/10.1007/s00406-013.0436-x.

114. Schoepf et al., "Physical Comorbidity and Its Relevance on Mortality in Schizophrenia"; Chi-Shin Wu, Mei-Shu Lai, and Susan Shur-Fen Gau, "Complications and Mortality in Patients with Schizophrenia and Diabetes: Population-Based Cohort Study," *British Journal of Psychiatry* 207, no. 5 (2015): 450–457, https://doi.org/10.1192/bjp.bp.113.143925; and Chi-Shin Wu and Susan Shur-Fen Gau, "Associations between Antipsychotic Treatment and Advanced Diabetes Complications among Schizophrenia Patients with Type 2 Diabetes Mellitus," Schizophrenia Bulletin 42, no. 3 (2016): 703–711, https://doi.org/10.1093/schbul/sbv187.

115. Taryn Becker and Janet Hux, "Risk of Acute Complications of Diabetes among People with Schizophrenia in Ontario, Canada," *Diabetes Care* 34, no. 2 (2011): 398–402, https://doi.org/10.2337/dc10-1139.

116. Becker and Hux, "Risk of Acute Complications of Diabetes among People with Schizophrenia in Ontario, Canada."

117. Schoepf et al., "Physical Comorbidity and Its Relevance on Mortality in Schizophrenia."

118. Schoepf et al., "Physical Comorbidity and Its Relevance on Mortality in Schizophrenia."

119. Emily G. Severance et al., "Gastroenterology Issues in Schizophrenia: Why the Gut Matters," *Current Psychiatry Reports* 17, no. 27 (2015): 1–10, https://doi.org/10.1007/s11920-015-0574-0.

120. Severance et al., "Gastroenterology Issues in Schizophrenia."

121. E. Fuller Torrey and Robert H. Yolken, "Schizophrenia and Infection: The Eyes Have It," *Schizophrenia Bulletin* 43, no. 2 (2017): 247–252, https://doi.org/10.1093/schbul/sbw113.

122. American Optometric Association, "Nystagmus," retrieved March 10, 2018, https://www.aoa.org/patients-and-public/eye-and-vision-problems/glossary-of-eye-and-vision-conditions/nystagmus.

123. Torrey and Yolken, "Schizophrenia and Infection."

124. Torrey and Yolken, "Schizophrenia and Infection."

125. Torrey and Yolken, "Schizophrenia and Infection."

126. Killian A. Welch et al., "Systematic Review of the Clinical Presentation of Schizophrenia in Intellectual Disability," *Journal of Psychopathology and Behavioral Assessment* 33, no. 2 (2011): 246–253, https://doi.org/10.1007/s10862-011-9224-y.

7

Traumatic Brain Injury

You are dispatched for a 24-year-old male having a seizure. Upon your arrival, your patient, Sam, is no longer seizing but is slightly postictal and complaining of a severe headache that he says he has had most of the day. When you ask about medical history, Sam's mother says that he had a traumatic brain injury two years ago after being in a car accident and was in a coma for several days. Sam lives with chronic headaches and occasional seizures. This seizure lasted longer than his typical seizures, and coupled with his severe headache, a thorough medical evaluation is appropriate. You obtain IV access in case he has more seizures, but he remains stable and alert during transport.

EMS providers are trained early in their careers to assess and treat patients who have sustained traumatic brain injuries (TBIs). Providers know to look for signs of increased intracranial pressure with *Cushing's triad* (irregular breathing, bradycardia, and widening pulse pressure), decreased levels of consciousness or disorientation, irregular/unequal/unreactive pupils, vomiting, increased blood pressure, and so on. They know to stabilize and treat, and that the best place for a brain-injured patient to receive definitive care is at a trauma center. But what happens after the patients return home? Although many patients recover fully and have minimal or no long-lasting effects, others experience significant and permanent damage that can impact their lives in a variety of ways. The purpose of this chapter is not to review the assessment and treatment of brain injuries at the time of injury but to consider the impact of the long-term effects of traumatic brain injury, and the role of EMS in the assessment and treatment of patients with a history of previous traumatic brain injury.

Statistics

The Centers for Disease Control and Prevention reported approximately 2.5 million TBI-related emergency department visits, approximately 282,000 TBI-related hospitalizations, and approximately 56,000 TBI-related deaths in 2013.[1] This accounted for 1 of every 50 emergency department visits and 2.2% of all deaths in the United States in 2013. The highest numbers of emergency department visits and hospitalizations occurred in three age groups: older than 75 years, newborn to 4 years old, and 15 to 24 years old. The highest death rates occurred in the age groups above 55 years of age. The most common causes of traumatic brain injuries were falls, being hit by or against an object, and motor vehicle collisions, as well as self-harm and assault. Of those deaths attributed to self-inflicted injuries, the majority were in males (87%), and 97% of those deaths were caused by firearms.[2]

The US Department of Education reported 26,000 students between the ages of 3 and 21 years old received special education services for brain injuries during the 2013 to 2014 school year,[3] 10,000 more than those who received services in the 2000 to 2001 school year.

Brain Anatomy and Physiology

The human brain has three main sections: the *cerebrum*, the *cerebellum*, and the *brain stem* (fig. 7–1). There are 12 pairs of cranial nerves that originate or start in the brain and the brain stem and relay information to other parts of the body.[4]

Cerebrum

The *cerebrum* is the largest part of the brain and is divided into the left and right hemispheres and four lobes: frontal, temporal, parietal, and occipital. Although there can be overlap in the lobes when it comes to physiology, each lobe is generally responsible for specific functions as follows:

- *Frontal lobe.* Responsible for personality, judgement, decision making, memory integration, voluntary movement, language, speech, and the executive functions of metacognition, organization, and planning.

- *Temporal lobe.* Responsible for visual and verbal memory, speech, language, object and facial recognition, interpretation of emotion, and auditory and visual processing.

- *Parietal lobe.* Responsible for visual-spatial processing, touch recognition, processing pressure and pain.
- *Occipital lobe.* Responsible for visual processing, color/shape recognition and processing.

Cerebellum

The *cerebellum*, smaller than the cerebrum, is located beneath the occipital lobe and on top of the brainstem. It is responsible for coordinating voluntary motor movements, including posture, balance, coordination, and speech.

Brain stem

The *brain stem* connects the brain to the spinal cord and is comprised of the midbrain, pons, and medulla oblongata:

- *Midbrain.* Controls eye movement.
- *Pons.* Coordinates eye and facial movement, and balance.
- *Medulla oblongata.* Controls the autonomic nervous system, which regulates the life-sustaining functions of breathing (respiration and ventilation), blood pressure, heart muscle contractions and heart rate, digestion, reflexive vomiting, coughing, sneezing, and swallowing.

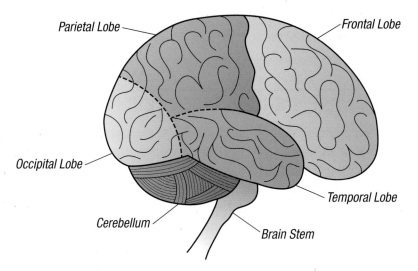

Fig. 7–1. Lobes of the brain

Cranial nerves

There are twelve cranial nerve pairs, and they serve specific functions as follows:

    I. *Olfactory.* Sense of smell.

    II. *Optic.* Transmission of visual input.

    III. *Oculomotor.* Eye movement, eyelid opening, and pupil dilation/constriction.

    IV. *Trochlear.* Eye movement.

    V. *Trigeminal.* Sensation to the face and muscles of chewing, motor innervation of extrinsic laryngeal muscles.

    VI. *Abducens.* Eye movement.

    VII. *Facial.* Eyelid closing, facial movement and expression, motor innervation of extrinsic laryngeal muscles.

    VIII. *Auditory/vestibular.* Hearing, balance through innervation of the semicircular canals in the ear.

    IX. *Glossopharyngeal.* Innervation of the salivary glands, oropharynx, tongue, and gag reflex.

    X. *Vagus.* Parasympathetic innervation controlling breathing, heart rate, and digestion as well as sensory and motor movement of the larynx.

    XI. *Accessory.* Neck and shoulder movement and strength.

    XII. *Hypoglossal.* Movement of the tongue and motor innervation of extrinsic laryngeal muscles.

What Is a Traumatic Brain Injury?

The Brain Injury Association of America (BIAA) defines a traumatic brain injury as "an alteration in brain function, or other evidence of brain pathology, caused by an external force" and differentiates it from an acquired brain injury that can occur from stroke, anoxia, hypoxia, cancer, illness, and the like.[5] The location of the injury, the area of the brain damaged, and the severity of the injury will determine what type of deficits the patient might experience post-injury.

The BIAA describes a variety of different types of traumatic brain injuries that can cause problems that linger beyond the original injury.[6]

- *Diffuse axonal injury.* This type of injury is caused when there have been shaking or rotational forces of the head, and the movement of the brain is unable to keep up with the movement of the skull. This results in swelling, shearing, and/or tearing of nerve tissues (axons) and can lead to widespread damage, coma, or death. The mortality rate of this type of injury may be as high as 62%.[7] Patients with a diffuse axonal injury can have long-term, debilitating injuries.

- *Concussion.* This is the most common type of traumatic brain injury[8] and may be caused by a blow to the head, shaking of the head, or whiplash. The person may briefly lose consciousness after the injury or may remain conscious but feel dazed afterward.

- *Contusion.* A contusion, or bruise, is the result of a blow to the head and can cause bleeding within the brain.

- *Second impact syndrome.* This type of traumatic brain injury occurs shortly after an initial injury and before that original injury has healed completely. This can cause cumulative, and sometimes severe, damage. Individuals with a recent head injury are at greater risk for a second injury.

- *Penetrating injury.* A penetrating injury occurs when a bullet or other sharp object goes through the skull into the brain, causing damage not only from the impact but also from the collateral damage from bone, skin, hair, and dirt and debris traveling inside the brain in addition to the penetrating object. Secondary damage occurs due to shearing, swelling, and bleeding of brain tissue.

- *Shaken baby syndrome.* This devastating and entirely preventable act happens when a parent or caregiver shakes a baby or toddler, usually in an effort to quiet their crying. This can cause diffuse axonal injuries, contusions, swelling, and bleeding. The effects of shaken baby syndrome can be significant, severe, long-lasting, and possibly fatal.

Concussions

Concussions are typically considered a mild traumatic brain injury, and it is therefore sometimes assumed that they are of little long-term consequence. This is a dangerous assumption, as concussions can take months to years to heal completely and have long-term effects. Researchers looking at the long-term effects of concussions found patients still experiencing debilitating symptoms as long as 11 years after the injury. The most common symptoms were fatigue, both mental and physical, headache, and poor memory.[9] Other studies support those findings, as well as increased incidence of depression, anxiety, mild cognitive impairment, and, rarely, suicide.[10]

Because the acute symptoms of a concussion can persist for several days post-injury, EMS providers should be aware of this and be prepared to assess accordingly if their patient reports a recent mild head injury and ongoing or new symptoms that could be related to a concussion.

Craton, Ali, and Lenoski describe an assessment tool for primary care providers to use when assessing a patient with a possible concussion to help facilitate a thorough evaluation.[11] Although this tool is designed for an "office-based assessment,"[12] its components can be useful for EMS providers in the field as they assess patients with a recent history of head injuries who are still experiencing problems. An acronym, COACH-CV, can help providers remember the components.

C—*Cognitive.* Cognitive difficulties include problems with alertness, orientation, memory, attention, concentration, processing speed, etc. Alertness and orientation can be assessed through the Glasgow Coma Scale (GCS), documenting if the patient is alert, responsive to verbal or painful stimuli, or unresponsive (AVPU), and/or the standard questions to assess if a patient is oriented to person, place, and time. Other cognitive difficulties may be ascertained by patient and/or family member report.

O—*Oculomotor manifestations.* This can include unusual eye movements, sensitivity to light, blurred vision, and headaches.

A—*Affective disturbances.* Affective symptoms can include depression, fatigue, sadness, irritability, poor sleep, and anxiety.

C—*Cervical pain.* While a concussion itself will not cause neck or cervical pain, there is an overlap between concussions and whiplash, so patients with a concussion may also experience neck pain that can be severe.

H—*Headaches.* Headaches, including migraine and tension headaches, are the most common post-concussion symptom, especially in people who already have a history of headaches.

C—*Cardiovascular manifestations.* Lesser well-known effects of concussions are problems with elevated heart rate, irregular heart rate, postural orthostatic tachycardia, and exercise intolerance. Be sure to assess vital signs carefully in post-concussion patients, including orthostatic vital signs in patients complaining of dizziness and lightheadedness.

V—*Vestibular dysfunction.* The majority of post-concussion patients can display vestibular dysfunction, including problems with balance, vertigo, and walking. Be cautious when moving patients who have had a concussion and are complaining of vestibular symptoms, especially when they are walking independently, to make sure they do not fall and cause a new injury or exacerbate the current one.

Defining severity

At the time of injury, EMS and receiving hospital providers will typically calculate a patient's Glasgow Coma Scale (table 7–1). A GCS of less than 8 points is considered a severe injury, 9–12 is a moderate injury, and 12–15 is a mild injury. It is important to note, however, that initial severity does not always correlate to prognosis. Although most people with mild injuries recover completely, their recovery can be long, and there can be long-lasting symptoms or deficits. Conversely, some people with severe injuries can make full recoveries over time.

Table 7–1. Glasgow Coma Scale

Glasgow Coma Scale		
Eye opening	Spontaneous opening	4
	Opening to verbal command/stimulus	3
	Opening to painful stimulus	2
	Does not open	1
Verbal response	Oriented and converses	5
	Disoriented/confused but converses	4
	Inappropriate responses	3
	Incomprehensive speech/sounds	2
	No verbal response	1
Motor response	Obeys commands to move	6
	Localizes pain/purposeful movement to pain	5
	Withdraws from pain	4
	Abnormal flexion to pain (decorticate posturing)	3
	Extension to pain (decerebrate posturing)	2
	No motor response	1

The American Psychiatric Association, in the *Diagnostic and Statistical Manual of Mental Disorders*,[13] provides three injury characteristics that can be rated to determine initial injury severity but also notes that initial injury severity does not necessarily correlate with long-term prognosis or outcome (table 7–2).

Table 7–2. Traumatic brain injury severity

Traumatic Brain Injury Severity			
Sign/symptom	Mild injury	Moderate injury	Severe injury
Loss of consciousness	Less than 30 minutes	Up to 24 hours	Greater than 24 hours
Memory loss after the injury	Less than 24 hours	24 hours to 7 days	Greater than 7 days
Glasgow Coma Scale at the time of injury	13–15 (not less than 13 at 30 minutes post-injury)	9–12	3–8

Source: Adapted from APA, *Diagnostic and Statistical Manual of Mental Disorders* (DSM-5), 626.

Common Cognitive Deficits after Traumatic Brain Injury

The most obvious and challenging deficits after a brain injury are cognitive changes in the areas of attention, learning/memory, executive functioning, and language/communication (table 7–3).[14] These deficits can resolve within a couple of months after the initial injury, or they can persist in varying degrees of severity.

Table 7–3. Possible deficits following a brain injury

Possible Deficits Following a Brain Injury

Area of deficit	Possible difficulties or characteristics*	Implications for EMS
Attention	• *Arousal and general alertness* to sensory input and difficulty responding appropriately to that input • *Sustained attention*, or the ability to maintain attention over time • *Selective attention*, or the ability to attend to a desired stimulus and ignore extraneous or irrelevant stimuli • *Processing speed*, or the time needed to process cognitive information, make decisions, or answer questions	Patients may have trouble with: • Attending to questions posed by EMS providers. • Answering questions quickly, accurately, and relevantly. • Focusing during a noisy, crowded, or brightly lit scene.
Learning/ memory	• *Declarative memory*, or the ability to remember events and facts • *Implicit memory*, or unconscious memory built on past experiences • *Working memory*, or the ability to hold small amounts of information in memory to be able to use it • *Prospective memory*, or remembering what one intends to do in the future • *Metamemory*, or recognizing that one has memory deficits and understanding the severity of those deficits	Patients may have trouble with: • Being able to recall events leading up to an emergency situation (why they called 911, how long they have had pain, how they acquired a new injury, if they took prescribed medication, etc.). • Remembering to go to routine or follow-up medical appointments, taking prescribed medication, checking blood sugar, etc.
Executive functioning	• Establishing and following through on goals and plans • Anticipating potential outcomes or consequences • Flexibility in thinking • Inhibition of behaviors • Reasoning and judgment • Problem solving • Impulsive language and behaviors	Patients may have trouble with: • Not being able to adequately consider negative consequences, exhibit good judgment in decision making, or inhibit impulsive words or behaviors can contribute to behaviors that can lead to the need for EMS.

Table 7–3. ...*continued*

| Speech/ language/ commu- nication/ literacy | • *Aphasia*, or difficulties understanding or producing spoken language, including issues with word recall, correct word usage/ semantics, correct grammar/ syntax
• *Alexia*, or difficulties with reading or recognizing the written word
• *Agraphia*, or problems with producing writing
• *Apraxia*, or speech difficulties, including impaired fluency, articulation (incorrect production of speech sounds), or coordination of speech production
• *Pragmatics*, or the social aspect of language, being able to read body language, facial expressions, tone of voice, initiating and maintaining conversations | • Patients may be unable to understand questions posed by providers or may be unable to find the words needed to express their answers.
• Impaired word finding, usage, and order within a sentence as well as impaired articulation or fluency may impede the EMS provider's understanding of the patient and can have a detrimental impact on assessment and treatment.
• Patients who are unable to read may not understand or follow written treatment orders which can lead to gaps in medical care and necessitate an EMS response.
• Patients who are unable to read also may not take prescription medication properly. They may underdose or overdose, each potentially creating a medical emergency.
• Having trouble with pragmatic or nonverbal language can lead to frustration, confusion, or communication breakdown on both sides of the conversation. |

Source: *Adapted from Silver, McAllister, and Yudofsky, *Textbook of Traumatic Brain Injury.*

Common Neuropsychiatric Deficits after Traumatic Brain Injury

Patients with a traumatic brain injury can experience psychiatric symptoms in the weeks, months, and years following the onset of injury. Patients can have delirium, depression, mood instability, psychosis, anxiety, post-traumatic stress disorder, changes in personality, and aggression (table 7–4).[15]

Table 7–4. Common neuropsychiatric deficits following traumatic brain injury

Common Neuropsychiatric Deficits Following Traumatic Brain Injury

Area of deficit	Possible difficulties/characteristics*	Implications for EMS
Delirium	• Disorientation • Disorganized, rambling thinking • Delusions • Disturbances in perception such as hallucinations • Sleep-wake cycle disturbances • Unstable mood • Problems with word choice/use	• Patients may be confused, incoherent, or disoriented. • Their behaviors can be worrisome to family and bystanders and can elicit a law enforcement response. • Patients may exhibit aggressive behaviors.

Mood instability	• Depression
	  – Depressed, sad, or irritable mood
	  – Sleeping too much or not enough
	  – Poor concentration
	  – Increased risk of suicide
	• Mania†
	  – Minimal sleep
	  – Pressured/rapid speech
	  – Delusions of grandeur
	  – Racing thoughts
	  – Participation in activities that are potentially dangerous or lead to negative consequences
		• Increased risk of alcohol or substance use or overdose can lead to an EMS response.
		• Brain injury can elevate the effects of psychiatric medications so side effects can be greater than anticipated.
		• Suicidal ideation or attempts can lead to an EMS response.
		• Pressured or rapid speech may make assessment difficult.
		• Poor judgment can lead to behavior that is inherently dangerous or puts the person in situations that are dangerous, subsequently creating the need for an EMS response.

Psychosis, including schizophrenia	• Auditory or visual hallucinations • Delusions† • Beliefs that do not change despite clear evidence to the contrary. • Delusions can be a belief in being persecuted or harmed or a belief in having exceptional abilities, wealth, or power.	• Psychotic patients can be difficult to assess and treat. They may not allow EMS providers to touch them or conduct assessments for fear that they will be harmed. • They may believe they are indestructible and are not ill or injured even when it appears obvious. • Their hallucinations or delusions may place them in situations where they are at increased risk of harm.

Table 7–4. ...*continued*

Anxiety	• Excessive worry accompanied by restlessness, fatigue, poor concentration, irritability, and/or sleep disturbances[†] • New onset of obsessive-compulsive disorder, post-traumatic stress disorder, generalized anxiety disorder.	• Patients may call 911 frequently for minor complaints. • They may be hard to convince that minor issues are indeed minor. • Conversely, they may have concerns or worry about possible treatment or transport to the hospital and may need to be convinced they need medical treatment.
Personality changes	• Regression to childish behavior. • Behavior inappropriate to the situation/poor judgment. • Aggression and irritability. • Mood instability or poor mood control.	• There may be increased difficulty with assessment. • Patients may be hostile, irritable, or unwilling to communicate with EMS or family members.
Aggression/ violence	• *Reactive*—Triggered by minor issue. • *Nonreflective*—Not planned or premeditated. • *Nonpurposeful*—Appears to serve no purpose. • *Explosive*—No buildup, comes out of nowhere. • *Periodic*—Brief outbursts with long periods of calm.[††]	• Scene safety is an EMS priority. • May be exacerbated by alcohol or drug use. • Consider the need for chemical sedation. • Utilize de-escalation techniques (as explained in chapter 1).

Sources:

[*]Adapted from Silver, McAllister, and Yudofsky, *Textbook of Traumatic Brain Injury*; and Ahmed et al., "Traumatic Brain Injury and Neuropsychiatric Complications."

[†]American Psychiatric Association, *Diagnostic and Statistical Manual of Mental Disorders*, 5th ed.

[††]Adapted from Silver, McAllister, and Yudofsky, *Textbook of Traumatic Brain Injury*, 261; and Ahmed et al., "Traumatic Brain Injury and Neuropsychiatric Complications."

Other Common Post-Injury Complications

Seizures

Seizures, or *post-traumatic epilepsy*, can be a common secondary effect of a traumatic brain injury, especially with a severe brain injury.[16] Seizures can occur in 5% to 7% of people hospitalized with a traumatic brain injury.[17] Risk of post-traumatic seizures is high in the pediatric population, occurring in as many as 12% of children with closed-head injuries and 50% of children with penetrating injuries.[18] The presence of post-traumatic seizures can have a negative impact on long-term prognosis due to the complications from the seizures themselves, such as hypoxia, increased intracranial pressure, and metabolic demands.[19] Post-traumatic seizures can also worsen cognitive and behavioral deficits created by the initial injury.[20]

Torbic et al. note factors for increased seizure risk after a traumatic brain injury.[21] Risk factors for early (less than seven days after injury) post-traumatic seizures include the following:

- GCS <10 at the time of original injury
- Seizures at the time of injury
- Penetrating injury
- Severe injury
- Linear or depressed skull fracture
- Alcoholism
- Post-injury amnesia lasting less than 30 minutes
- Subdural, epidural, or intracerebral hematoma
- Younger than 65 years of age

Risk factors for late (greater than seven days after injury) seizures include:

- Early post-traumatic seizures
- Intracerebral hematoma
- Severe injury
- Post-injury amnesia lasting longer than 24 hours
- Loss of consciousness at the time of injury
- Older than 65 years of age

Some post-brain injury seizures may be prevented with anti-seizure medications, but there is discussion concerning whether or not all patients with a history of traumatic brain injury should be treated prophylactically with anti-seizure medications.[22] A review of the use of post-TBI prophylactic anti-seizure medications conducted by Torbic et al. suggests that these medications are beneficial during the first week post-injury.[23] Be sure to ask if your patient is taking anti-seizure medications.

Headache

Headache is one of the most common post-traumatic brain injury symptoms reported and can have a negative impact on quality of life.[24] Headache symptoms can take some time to resolve post-injury. In the study from Hong et al. of 259 patients with a traumatic brain injury who reported a new onset of headache following injury, 40% still reported moderate to severe headaches 12 months after their injury, and 13% (those who had post-traumatic seizure and intracranial hemorrhage) reported moderate to severe headaches 36 months post-injury.[25] When assessing patients with a history of traumatic brain injury and headache, be sure to conduct a thorough assessment, including a stroke scale, to rule out other sources of the headache.

Substance use/abuse

The association between substance abuse and traumatic brain injury is twofold. People with a history of alcohol or drug abuse are at higher risk for sustaining a traumatic brain injury due to risky behaviors associated with substance abuse[26] and may be at risk for greater damage as a result of an injury than those who are not heavy drinkers prior to a traumatic brain injury.[27] Ongoing substance abuse can have a negative impact on recovery. Alcohol use following a traumatic brain injury can increase the risk for seizures, subsequent injuries, cognitive deficits, and emotional and behavioral difficulties.[28] Chronic alcoholism can cause brain tissue atrophy, which can complicate recovery and increase limitations following injury.[29]

People who have a history of traumatic brain injury may be at a greater risk for new or exacerbated substance use following the injury, although the evidence is inconclusive.[30]

Implications for EMS

The long-term complications following a traumatic brain injury can be complex and can include physical, psychiatric, and cognitive challenges. When assessing a patient who has a history of a traumatic brain injury, you will want to consider the following while conducting your assessment:

- Length of time since the injury
- Location of the injury
- Type (open, closed, penetrating)

- Any known complications
- Any history of seizures, either immediately post-injury or currently

When speaking with your patient, conduct your assessment as you would with any other patient, while keeping in mind that they may have cognitive or psychiatric issues that are not obvious or may become exacerbated during a stressful emergency.

Be prepared for the following:

- Confusion or disorientation
- Difficulty answering questions
- Poor memory, both of events and personal history
- Aggression or behavioral issues
- Pain management (headaches)
- Seizures

Notes

1. Christopher A. Taylor et al., "Traumatic Brain Injury–Related Emergency Department Visits, Hospitalizations, and Deaths—United States, 2007 and 2013," *Morbidity and Mortality Weekly Report: Surveillance Summaries* 66, no. 9 (2017): 1–20, https://doi.org/10.15585/mmwr.ss6609a1.

2. Taylor et al., "Traumatic Brain Injury–Related Emergency Department Visits, Hospitalizations, and Deaths."

3. US Department of Education, Institute of Educational Sciences, National Center for Education Statistics, *Digest of Education Statistics*, 2015 (NCES 2016-014), chapter 2 (Washington, DC: US Dept. of Education, IES, NCES, 2016), retrieved from https://nces.ed.gov/fastfacts/display.asp?id=64.

4. American Association of Neurological Surgeons, "Anatomy of the Brain," 2017, retrieved October 21, 2017, http://www.aans.org/Patients/Neurosurgical-Conditions-and-Treatments/Anatomy-of-the-Brain.

5. Brain Injury Association of America, "About Brain Injury: Brain Injury Overview," retrieved October 15, 2017, from http://www.biausa.org/about-brain-injury.htm.

6. Brain Injury Association of America, "About Brain Injury."

7. Junwei Ma et al., "Progress of Research on Diffuse Axonal Injury after Traumatic Brain Injury," *Neural Plasticity* (2016): 1–7, https://doi.org/10.1155/2016/9746313.

8. Saeed Ahmed et al., "Traumatic Brain Injury and Neuropsychiatric Complications," *Indian Journal of Psychological Medicine* 39, no. 2 (2017): 114–121, https://doi.org/10.4103/0253-7176.203129.

9. Sara Åhman et al., "Long-Term Follow-up of Patients with Mild Traumatic Brain Injury: A Mixed-Method Study," *Journal of Rehabilitation Medicine* 45, no. 8 (2013): 758–764, https://doi.org/10.2340/16501977-1182.

10. Michael Fralick et al., "Risk of Suicide after a Concussion," *Canadian Medical Association Journal* 188, no. 7 (2016): 497–504, https://doi.org/10.1503/cmaj.150790; Philippe Decq et al., "Long-Term Consequences of Recurrent Sports Concussion," *Acta Neurochirurgica* 158, no. 2 (2015): 289–300, https://doi.org/10.1007/s00701-015-2681-4; and Natalie Sandel et al., "Anxiety and Mood Clinical Profile following Sport-Related Concussion: From Risk Factors to Treatment," *Sport, Exercise, and Performance Psychology* 6, no. 3 (2017): 304–323, https://doi.org/10.1037/spy0000098.

11. Neil Craton, Haitham Ali, and Stephane Lenoski, "COACH CV: The Seven Clinical Phenotypes of Concussion," *Brain Sciences* 7, no. 9 (2017): 119, https://doi.org/10.3390/brainsci7090119.

12. Craton, Ali, and Lenoski, "COACH CV," 1.

13. American Psychiatric Association, *Diagnostic and Statistical Manual of Mental Disorders*, 5th ed. (Washington, DC: APA, 2013).

14. Jonathan M. Silver, Thomas W. McAllister, and Stuart C. Yudofsky, eds. *Textbook of Traumatic Brain Injury* (Washington, DC: American Psychiatric Publishing, 2005).

15. Silver, McAllister, and Yudofsky, *Textbook of Traumatic Brain Injury*; and Ahmed et al., "Traumatic Brain Injury and Neuropsychiatric Complications."

16. David Chadwick, "Seizures and Epilepsy after Traumatic Brain Injury," *The Lancet*, 355, no. 9,201 (2000): 334–336, https://doi.org/10.1016/s0140-6736(99)00452-3; and Asla Pitkänen and Riikka Immonen, "Epilepsy Related to Traumatic Brain Injury," *Neurotherapeutics* 11, no. 2 (2014): 286–296, https://doi.org/10.1007/s13311-014-0260-7.

17. Heather Torbic et al., "Use of Antiepileptics for Seizure Prophylaxis after Traumatic Brain Injury," *American Journal of Health-System Pharmacy* 70, no. 9 (2013): 759–766, https://doi.org/10.2146/ajhp120203.

18. Jorge I. Arango et al., "Posttraumatic Seizures in Children with Severe Traumatic Brain Injury," *Child's Nervous System* 28, no. 11 (2012): 1,925–1,929, https://doi.org/10.1007/s00381-012-1863-0.

19. Arango et al., "Posttraumatic Seizures in Children with Severe Traumatic Brain Injury."

20. Arango et al., "Posttraumatic Seizures in Children with Severe Traumatic Brain Injury."

21. Torbic et al., "Use of Antiepileptics for Seizure Prophylaxis after Traumatic Brain Injury,"

22. Chadwick, "Seizures and Epilepsy after Traumatic Brain Injury."

23. Torbic et al., "Use of Antiepileptics for Seizure Prophylaxis after Traumatic Brain Injury."

24. Chang-Ki Hong et al., "The Course of Headache in Patients with Moderate-to-Severe Headache Due to Mild Traumatic Brain Injury: A Retrospective Cross-Sectional Study," *Journal of Headache and Pain* 18 (2017): 1–7, https://doi.org/10.1186/s10194-017-0755-9.

25. Hong et al., "The Course of Headache in Patients with Moderate-to-Severe Headache Due to Mild Traumatic Brain Injury."

26. Ahmed et al., "Traumatic Brain Injury and Neuropsychiatric Complications"; and Steven L. West, "Substance Use among Persons with Traumatic Brain Injury: A Review," *Neurorehabilitation* 29, no. 1 (2011): 1–8, https://doi.org/10.3233/NRE-2011-0671.

27. Jennie Ponsford, Laura Tweedly, and John Taffe, "The Relationship between Alcohol and Cognitive Functioning following Traumatic Brain Injury," *Journal of Clinical and Experimental Neuropsychology* 35, no. 1 (2013): 103–112, https://doi.org/10.1080/13803395.2012.752437.

28. Summar Reslan and Robin A. Hanks, "Factors Associated with Alcohol-Related Problems following Moderate to Severe Traumatic Brain Injury," *Rehabilitation Psychology* 59, no. 4 (2014): 453–458, https://doi.org/10.1037/a0037186.

29. West, "Substance Use among Persons with Traumatic Brain Injury."

30. Daniel F. Gros et al., "Co-Occurring Traumatic Brain Injury, PTSD Symptoms, and Alcohol Use in Veterans," *Journal of Psychopathology and Behavioral Assessment* 38, no. 2 (2016): 266–273, https://doi.org/10.1007/s10862-015-9513-y.

8

Special Medical Conditions

Alcohol Use Disorder

You are dispatched as an ALS chase vehicle to rendezvous with a BLS transport vehicle that is arriving on scene at a gated industrial complex. Upon arrival you are greeted by the security guards, who direct you to the patient, who is under the care of the EMTs. The guards state that the patient drove around the gate and barriers onto the complex and only stopped when barricaded by security vehicles. The patient, John, a man in his mid-50s, is handcuffed and leaning against his vehicle, arguing with the EMT. As you begin to speak with him, you notice an odor similar to that of an alcoholic beverage, even though it is late morning, and he appears to be somewhat confused and belligerent. His blood sugar and other vital signs are within expected parameters. John offers that he has not "had anything to drink since last night" as he is trying to quit drinking. He reluctantly agrees to transport and is helped to the stretcher. En route to the hospital for evaluation, John begins to seize, which you are able to bring under control with benzodiazepine, and he is admitted to the ED for observation and support during his continued withdrawal from alcohol.

Alcoholism, also called *alcohol use disorder*, is a prevalent, expensive, and serious condition that affects millions of Americans[1] and is a common reason for requiring an EMS response or admission to the emergency department. Frequent visits to the hospital for alcohol-related issues place a burden on resources, however. There are numerous valid and serious reasons for an emergency department visit (discussed in more detail below), by ambulance or not, but often people visit the emergency department for less serious or unnecessary reasons.[2]

Researchers who conducted a recent study in which they interviewed people with an alcohol use disorder[3] reported that while these individuals had many of the chronic or acute medical issues related to alcohol use, they also found that emergency departments were places where they could achieve any or all of the following:

1. Receive social support (such as meals, shelter from the elements, clean clothes)

2. Gain access to routine medical care they were otherwise unable to obtain due to lack of available resources or transportation

3. Allay fears that they might experience withdrawal symptoms by going to the emergency department preemptively

While these less-urgent reasons place a burden on both prehospital and hospital resources, the patients involved feel a genuine need to access care. Prehospital and hospital staff not only can provide some of this care, they can also help patients access additional resources as appropriate.

What is an alcohol use disorder?

According to the Center for Behavioral Health Statistics and Quality, in 2014 there were 60.9 million Americans 12 years and older who reported binge alcohol use in the previous month, and of those binge drinkers, 16.3 million reported heavy alcohol use in the previous month.[4] Binge alcohol use and heavy alcohol use are defined as follows:

- *Binge alcohol use.* Drinking five or more drinks on the same occasion on at least one day in the past 30 days.[5]

- *Heavy alcohol use.* Drinking five or more drinks on the same occasion on five or more days in the past 30 days.[6]

The Center for Behavioral Health Statistics and Quality also reported that of the 17 million people aged 12 or older in the United States with a diagnosis of an alcohol use disorder in 2014, 2.6 million of them also had a concurrent illicit drug use disorder.[7]

The American Psychiatric Association, in the fourth edition of their diagnostic manual, had two broad subcategories under their entry for alcohol use disorder called "alcohol dependence" and "alcohol abuse," with an additional entry for alcohol withdrawal.[8] The fifth edition of the diagnostic manual has one broad category encompassing dependence and abuse, and another category for withdrawal symptoms.[9]

The APA defines an *alcohol use disorder* as pattern of alcohol use that leads to impairment or distress, with *at least two* of the following symptoms within a 12-month period:[10]

- Alcohol is taken in larger amounts over a longer period than intended by the individual.

- A persistent desire to cut down or limit alcohol use that is often unsuccessful.

- A considerable amount of time is spent trying to obtain or use alcohol, or to recover from its effects

- A craving or urge to use alcohol.

- Recurrent alcohol use results in a failure to meet obligations at work, school, or home.

- Alcohol use continues despite having significant social or personal problems caused or worsened by the effects of alcohol.

- Social, occupational, or recreational activities are given up or limited because of alcohol use.

- Alcohol use continues in situations in which it is physically hazardous.

- Alcohol use continues despite the person knowing they have an ongoing physical or psychological problem likely to have been caused or worsened by alcohol use.

- Alcohol tolerance develops, including increased amounts of alcohol needed to reach intoxication or desired effect.

- The individual has withdrawal symptoms and may continue to drink or use another substance to reduce the withdrawal symptoms.

The severity of the alcohol use disorder is further clarified by the number of symptoms present:

- Mild: 2–3 symptoms
- Moderate: 4–5 symptoms
- Severe: 6 or more symptoms

Alcohol use disorders are associated with increased risk of illness, hospitalizations, and death, with one study reporting people with alcohol use disorders dying an average of 12 years younger than those without.[11] While men are more likely to abuse alcohol,[12] the risks may be higher for women than men. While women tend to consume less alcohol overall, differences in metabolism lead to greater blood concentrations of alcohol.[13] Alcohol may be responsible for almost 6% of deaths worldwide.[14] According to the Centers for Disease Control and Prevention, an average of more than 88,000 US deaths per year are attributable to chronic and acute excessive alcohol use.[15]

Most EMS providers are familiar with a typical call concerning a person who is under the influence of alcohol and is drunk. We know that excessive alcohol use can contribute to domestic violence, motor vehicle collisions, and other accidents. We are familiar with these patients being unsteady on their feet and perhaps stumbling and falling. We expect slurred speech and the possibility they may be belligerent or overly friendly and jovial. We are prepared for vomiting and to manage their airway if necessary. We may not, however, be aware of the potentially serious effects of chronic alcohol use that can complicate what might appear to be another routine call for a drunk person.

An alcohol use disorder can contribute to a number of ongoing medical issues such as liver disease, pancreatitis, excessive gastrointestinal bleeding, and thiamine deficiency (discussed in more detail below). Alcohol use disorder is also associated with an increased risk of cancer, stroke, non-withdrawal-related seizures, hypertension, and cardiovascular disease,[16] as well as increased comorbidity with psychiatric disorders such as depression and bipolar disorder.[17] Withdrawing from alcohol when dependent can cause its own set of serious health problems, such as nausea, vomiting, tremors, auditory/visual hallucinations, headache, disorientation, agitation/anxiety, and seizures (also discussed below). These collective symptoms are also called *delirium tremens* or *DTs*.[18]

Physical Symptoms of Alcohol Use Disorder

Liver disease

Liver damage and subsequent liver disease from alcohol use disorder are the primary contributors to liver disease in the United States[19] and have been reported as responsible for as many as two-thirds of alcohol-related deaths.[20] *Liver disease* includes the familiar *cirrhosis*, or scarring, of the liver, and also liver cancer. The risk of liver disease increases as the amount of alcohol ingested increases, and people who drink outside of meals increase their risk of liver disease by more than 2.5 times.[21] Alcohol-related liver disease can progress rapidly to alcohol hepatitis and/or liver cancer, which can lead to rapid liver failure and death.[22] Additionally, obesity increases the risk of developing liver disease or cirrhosis.[23]

Pancreatitis

Pancreatitis is a painful inflammation of the pancreas and is commonly associated with alcohol use disorder. While pancreatitis can have other causes, such as gallstones, alcohol use is the most common cause.[24]

Pancreatitis can be acute or chronic, and it can cause severe pain, dehydration, abdominal bleeding, and infection. Chronic pancreatitis can also lead to developing diabetes, malnutrition and food absorption problems, and pancreatic cancer.[25] In severe cases it can lead to death.[26]

Prehospital treatment for pancreatitis will mostly be symptom management, including fluids for dehydration, pain management, and blood glucose monitoring, with intervention as indicated.

Seizures

Seizures that occur during alcohol withdrawal are common, but people who are alcohol dependent are at an increased risk for seizures for other reasons related to the alcohol use. People with an alcohol use disorder are at increased risk (as much as three times) for developing a seizure disorder such as epilepsy.[27] People who misuse alcohol are at greater risk for head injuries, which can lead to seizures. Drug use concurrent with alcohol use can also cause seizures.

It is important to remember, however, that non-alcohol-related events such as withdrawal from other medications (such as benzodiazepines or anticonvulsants), brain tumors, strokes, and other illnesses can cause seizures, so do not assume that all seizures in people without a known seizure disorder are related to alcohol use.[28] Be sure to conduct a thorough assessment and physical exam to rule out other issues that might need to be addressed.

Excessive gastrointestinal bleeding

Excessive gastrointestinal bleeding may be related to the following:

- *Esophageal varices.* When blood flow from the liver is obstructed by liver disease, blood is rerouted from the larger blood vessels into smaller vessels near the esophagus that are not designed to carry large volumes of blood. When these small veins become swollen and fragile, they are called *esophageal varices.* These varices may rupture, causing substantial and life-threatening bleeding.[29] Patients with cirrhosis of the liver and a history of esophageal variceal bleeding have a four times higher risk of experiencing another episode of bleeding.[30]

- *Other upper gastrointestinal bleeding.* Alcohol use disorder can lead to other types of bleeding from the gastrointestinal tract.[31] One-fifth of people with gastrointestinal bleeding use alcohol excessively, and it is associated with an increased risk of repeated bleeding and death.
  - Episodic heavy drinking can increase the risk of bleeding from gastric and duodenal ulcers.
  - A tear in the tissue where the esophagus meets the stomach is called a *Mallory-Weiss tear* and can be caused by excessive vomiting associated with alcohol use and is a common cause of bleeding in people with alcohol use disorder.

Thiamine deficiency and Wernicke's encephalopathy

Chronic alcohol use disorder can cause a deficiency in vitamin B1, or thiamine.[32] Thiamine deficiency can be caused by inadequate nutrition associated with alcohol use disorder due to decreased absorption of thiamine from the intestinal tract. Thiamine is needed by the body and brain for metabolizing glucose and carbohydrates.

A triad of symptoms is present in Wernicke's encephalopathy: encephalopathy, ataxic gait, and oculomotor dysfunction.[33]

- *Encephalopathy* is manifested by confusion, agitation, and other changes in mental status.
- *Ataxic gait* is manifested by walking very slowly with a wide stance, poor balance, or being unable to walk at all.
- *Oculomotor dysfunction* includes nystagmus, slow pupil responses, and changes in gaze.

In some cases, Wernicke's encephalopathy can lead to hypothermia, hypotension, heart failure, and coma.[34]

Prehospital interventions for Wernicke's encephalopathy include assessment and management of blood glucose levels, fluid replacement, and management of hypothermia and hypotension.[35]

Withdrawal symptoms

Symptoms of alcohol-dependence withdrawal include tachypnea, tachycardia, diaphoresis, irritability, hypertension, tremor, hallucinations, and seizures[36] and can start 6 to 24 hours after the last consumption of alcohol.[37]

Without appropriate treatment for mild or moderate alcohol withdrawal, the patient can experience delirium tremens, which can be serious. Symptoms of delirium tremens include hyperthermia, tachycardia, tachypnea, agitation, disorientation, hallucinations, and loss of consciousness.[38] Patients in this stage of withdrawal need hospital support.[39] Delirium tremens may occur in as many as 20% of people who are withdrawing from alcohol, and mortality rates may be as high as 15%.[40]

Seizures are one of the most serious complications associated with alcohol withdrawal and can appear as early as 6 hours (and up to 48 hours) after a person's last drink.[41] Alcohol can actually raise the seizure threshold in the brain, which is rapidly decreased when the depressant action on the brain is removed.[42] Seizures occur as the blood alcohol levels approach zero but can also occur when blood alcohol levels drop quickly while there is still alcohol in the blood. Thus a person who is still intoxicated can have a withdrawal-related seizure.[43]

Implications for EMS

- Try to suspend your judgment of the patient's drinking and treat the medical symptoms that are presenting. While early drinking may have been a choice, the alcohol-dependent patient has moved beyond the "choice" to drink and needs care and compassion when they are in crisis or withdrawal.

- Do not neglect to assess for other causes of unusual behaviors that may mimic intoxication, and do not forget to do a complete assessment for other potentially serious signs and symptoms either caused by the intoxication or masked or hidden by it. Be careful not to assume every presenting problem is attributable to "just being drunk."

- If there is an indication of esophageal variceal bleeding, especially if the patient has a history of such bleeding, be prepared to aggressively manage their airway and address hypovolemia from blood loss.

- Consider Wernicke's encephalopathy in any patient with a history of alcohol use disorder and significant neurological symptoms, especially if poor nutrition is also suspected. *Do not assume that an altered mental status or balance problems are due to the alcohol alone.* Be prepared to manage their airway, check blood glucose levels and treat accordingly, and manage hypotension and hypothermia. Administer IV thiamine with the glucose if your jurisdictional protocols allow.

- In patients with withdrawal symptoms, be prepared to manage seizures with airway support and benzodiazepines,[44] as they can happen suddenly, and be prepared for repeat seizures.

- Consider other reasons for seizures such as injury, hypoglycemia, medication withdrawal (or overdose), or established seizure disorder.

Cystic Fibrosis

You arrive on scene after a dispatch for a 17-year-old female with difficulty breathing. The patient, Anna, is well known to your crew as she has cystic fibrosis and you have transported her before. Today she looks unwell, with labored, rapid breathing. She is also tachycardic and febrile. Her blood pressure is in the low-normal range, and she is hypocapnic. Based on her symptoms and her high risk for infection, you suspect Anna has sepsis. You place her on supplemental oxygen, obtain IV access, start her on fluids per your sepsis protocol, and prepare for rapid transport to the emergency department, while also being prepared for the possibility of respiratory failure.

Cystic fibrosis is an inherited, chronic, progressive disease caused by a defective gene on chromosome 7 inherited from one or both parents.[45] The Cystic Fibrosis Foundation (CFF) reported in 2014 that there were more than

26,000 people living with cystic fibrosis in the United States.[46] Just under 900 new cases were reported that year, with more than 60% being diagnosed by newborn screening.[47]

Cystic fibrosis causes the body to produce an excess of thick, sticky mucus that is difficult to eliminate and subsequently builds up in the body, having a negative impact on several systems, especially the respiratory, gastrointestinal, and endocrine systems.[48]

The excess mucus builds up in the lungs, blocking the bronchioles and alveoli, causing chronic respiratory problems, difficulty breathing, and lung damage. It can also trap bacteria in the lungs and lead to respiratory infections. The mucus also impacts the gastrointestinal system by blocking the release of pancreatic and other digestive enzymes that digest food causing pancreatitis, and by interfering with the production of insulin, leading to diabetes. Liver involvement, potentially leading to cirrhosis, is seen as well. There is also an increased risk of osteoporosis and osteopenia due to vitamin D deficiency.[49]

People with cystic fibrosis have a variety of symptoms including a chronic (dry or productive) cough, frequent respiratory infections that can be drug resistant, poor weight gain or failure to thrive, diabetes, and a shortened life expectancy. The survival rate to adulthood has increased, with a median survival age of approximately 40 years (a 10-year gain since 1999), with more than 50% of patients currently over 18 years of age.[50] Although people with cystic fibrosis are living longer than ever, there is still a very high rate of hospital admissions, including ICU admissions with ventilation support.[51]

People who live in poverty have a poorer prognosis when living with cystic fibrosis. Circumstances that are common in poverty, such as insufficient access to proper nutrition, exposure to cigarette smoke, exposure to infections, and family stress, are more prevalent in families of low socioeconomic status.[52]

Lung disease

Lung disease is the most common cause of death in people with cystic fibrosis.[53] Ranganathan et al. describe four ways cystic fibrosis can impact a person's lungs and other pulmonary structures:[54]

- *Pulmonary inflammation.* Pulmonary inflammation starts as early as the first weeks of life and is associated with poor nutritional status, infection, and *bronchiectasis*, a condition in which the bronchioles are widened, thickened, and scarred, eventually becoming unable to remove mucous.[55]

- *Infection.* The most common bacteria cultured from patients with cystic fibrosis are *Staphylococcus aureus, Haemophilus influenzae,* and *Pseudomonas aeruginosa.* Infection is seen in early life, and the prevalence of infection increases with age. Because of the frequent respiratory infections, antibiotic use (inhaled, oral, and intravenous) is common, including prophylactic use of antibiotics to prevent infection.[56] *P. aeruginosa,* however, has been found to be particularly resistant to antibiotics, and its presence may be indicative of a more severe disease.[57]

- *Structural lung disease.* Chronic infection and inflammation can lead to bronchiectasis and subsequent irreversible damage to lung structures.

- *Lung function.* Lung function is diminished, and functionality can worsen with infection and inflammation.

Treatment for the chronic lung disease associated with cystic fibrosis is extensive, life-long, and multifaceted. Treatments include inhaled bronchodilators (albuterol/ipratropium), CPAP, antibiotics, chest therapy to loosen and expel trapped mucus, corticosteroids to reduce inflammation, oxygen, nutritional support, and lung transplant.[58] Exercise has also shown to be beneficial as it increases aerobic capacity and removal of mucus.[59]

Diabetes

Cystic fibrosis–related diabetes is reported to be the most common comorbidity in people with cystic fibrosis and is associated with an increased risk of death.[60] Women with cystic fibrosis are at a slightly higher risk for developing diabetes.

Although cystic fibrosis–related diabetes shares features with type I and type II diabetes, its origins are different.[61] Type I diabetes is autoimmune in nature and results in the destruction of beta cells in the pancreas that produce insulin. Type II diabetes comes from an acquired insulin resistance.[62] Diabetes related to cystic fibrosis, however, occurs when the pancreas is damaged through inflammation and obstruction.[63] This causes scarring, which decreases the ability of the pancreas to produce insulin. As the course of cystic fibrosis progresses and worsens, so can the manifestation of the diabetes. In addition, the effects of acute illness and corticosteroid use so prevalent in the cystic fibrosis population can exacerbate insulin resistance. Treatment for cystic fibrosis–related diabetes is similar to both type I and type II diabetes, a combination of insulin and, less frequently, oral medication.[64]

Gastrointestinal problems

Gastrointestinal problems are also common with people with cystic fibrosis. Tabori et al. report a number of pain-related and non-pain-related symptoms:[65]

- *Pain.* Abdominal pain can be experienced in all abdominal regions, but the most common areas are umbilical and epigastric. Many people report pain in more than one area, occurring as frequently as once per week, and lasting for several hours. Children report more abdominal pain symptoms than adults.

- *Non-pain-related symptoms.* These can include constipation, flatulence/gas, distension, nausea, vomiting, reflux, and heartburn.[66] These symptoms occur in similar frequency between children and adults except for abdominal distension and heartburn, which are more commonly reported by adults. Bulky, foul-smelling stools, poor appetite, or a large appetite with minimal or no weight gain can also occur.[67]

Nutrition

Children with cystic fibrosis frequently have issues with malnutrition, which can lead to stunted growth.[68] Poor growth in infants can be an early symptom leading to diagnosis. Malnutrition in these patients is caused by malabsorption of nutrients, increased energy output, and decreased caloric input.[69] Gastroesophageal reflux, prevalent in people with cystic fibrosis, is a common cause of malnutrition.[70]

Sleep disturbances

Children with cystic fibrosis have been reported to have sleep disturbances that can have a negative impact on their overall health. Children with cystic fibrosis were reported to have a later onset of sleep, an earlier waking time, and disordered breathing while sleeping. Health quality and sleep quality are correlated. Children with cystic fibrosis who had poorer sleep were perceived to be less healthy than those with cystic fibrosis with better sleep.[71]

Implications for EMS

- Minimize the patient's exposure to germs. Be sure to wear gloves and change them frequently. Wear a face mask if you have a cold or other illness.
- Remember to check blood glucose levels and treat accordingly.
- Consider pain management for severe abdominal pain.
- Patients in a respiratory crisis due to excessive mucus or other respiratory complications may need aggressive airway management. This can include medication therapy including nebulizer treatments (albuterol and ipratropium), CPAP, suctioning, manual ventilation by bag-valve mask, or intubation.[72]

PANDAS/PANS

You are responding for a seven-year-old female with a psychiatric emergency. The scene has been secured by law enforcement, so you proceed in. You enter the residence and see that the room has been destroyed. Chairs are overturned, newspapers and magazines are ripped and thrown around, all the toys are pulled off the shelf, and several boxes of puzzles are poured out. Your patient, Torie, is curled up on the couch with her face in the cushions. She is breathing heavily but seems calm. Her mom looks completely overwhelmed at the events. She has scratch marks and bruises on her arms but says she does not need medical attention.

Torie's mom says that Torie has never acted like this before. The mom did not know what to do other than call 911. You ask about medical history, and Torie's mom says she has no medical issues other than a history of strep throat, which was treated by antibiotics. As you approach Torie to assess her, she climbs on her mom's lap but allows you to take her vitals, including blood sugar, all of which are all within expected parameters. You ask her mom to get a couple of books and a favorite stuffed animal so Torie has something familiar in the ambulance. You go to the hospital with Torie and her mom for medical and psychiatric evaluations.

Pediatric Autoimmune Neuropsychiatric Disorders Associated with Streptococcal Infections (PANDAS), although in the literature since the 1990s, is an uncommon pediatric autoimmune disorder associated with a rapid onset of or worsening of obsessive-compulsive behaviors and/or vocal and/or motor tics following a streptococcal infection (such as strep throat or scarlet fever).[73] *Pediatric Acute-Onset Neuropsychiatric Syndrome (PANS)* is a disorder with the same rapid onset of behavioral symptoms without strep or any other known trigger.[74] Typical age of onset is between 3 and 12 years, and the average age of onset for PANDAS is 2 to 3 years younger than the average age of onset for childhood onset of obsessive-compulsive disorder and tic disorder.[75]

PANDAS/PANS is a diagnosis of exclusion; that is, there is nothing else that better explains the symptoms and behaviors.[76] The diagnostic criteria are listed in table 8–1.[77] Additional symptoms include food refusal, anxiety, emotional instability, inattention, hyperactivity, oppositional behaviors, behavioral regression, deteriorating handwriting, and psychosis.[78] The symptoms can appear very quickly (described as "lightning-like"[79]), even overnight, following a strep infection, and can be worsened by stress.[80] The onset of these symptoms, which can be sudden and severe, can be frightening to children and their parents, possibly resulting in a 911 call for transport to the hospital. Other proposed triggers for PANDAS/PANS include respiratory infections (such as mycoplasma pneumonia and influenza), Lyme disease, herpes simplex, and enterovirus.[81]

Table 8–1. Diagnostic criteria for PANDAS

Diagnostic Criteria for PANDAS
• Presence of obsessive-compulsive disorder and/or a tic disorder
• Pediatric onset of symptoms (age 3 years to puberty)
• Episodic course of symptom severity
• Association with group A beta-hemolytic streptococcal infection (a positive throat culture for strep or history of scarlet fever)
• Association with neurological abnormalities (physical hyperactivity or unusual, jerky movements that are not in the child's control)
• Very abrupt onset or worsening of symptoms

Source: US Dept. of HHS, NIH, NIMH, *PANDAS—Questions and Answers.*

PANDAS/PANS, as a diagnosis, was historically controversial due to limited research and difficulty clearly linking strep infections as a cause (rather than a correlation) of mental health and behavioral symptoms,[82] but a recent study published in *JAMA Psychiatry* reported that children with both streptococcal throat infections as well as non-streptococcal throat infections had a small, but increased, risk of mental health disorders, obsessive-compulsive disorder, and tic disorders.[83]

Several of the behaviors exhibited by children with PANDAS/PANS can pose a risk to their safety, so when assessing a patient with known or suspected PANDAS/PANS, be sure to be cognizant of these issues and be prepared to address them during transport. They include the following:[84]

- A history of physical violence or aggression, posing a danger to self or others

- Suicidal ideation

- Refusal to eat or drink, which can lead to malnutrition and dehydration

Treatment for children with PANDAS/PANS is multi-faceted and involves symptom management, removing the source of infection, and addressing immune deficiencies.[85] Treatment can include antibiotics to treat an active infection, prophylactic antibiotics, and intravenous immunoglobulin.[86] Some research provides initial support for tonsillectomy as a way to reduce the severity of symptoms in children diagnosed with PANDAS/PANS. Cognitive behavioral therapy can be utilized to reduce tics and other behavior issues, and psychiatric medications such as SSRIs and atypical antipsychotics have been effective.[87]

While EMS is not equipped to treat the underlying issues surrounding PANDAS/PANS, you may be called to treat a child with a new onset of symptoms that are concerning to a parent or caregiver, or the child could be in a behavioral or psychiatric crisis related to the PANDAS/PANS diagnosis.

Implications for EMS

- Keep the patient safe from self-harm. Consider physical restraint or chemical sedation as a last resort and only if the patient is a danger to self or others. Severe behaviors may need to be controlled with benzodiazepines if allowed in your local protocols for behavior emergencies.[88] Some medications, especially antipsychotics, used to treat PANDAS/PANS can cause a prolonged QTc, so be especially cautious before administering Haldol and obtain a 12-lead EKG before doing so.[89]

- This is a physical condition that presents with apparent mental health or behavioral symptoms (see chapter 6). If there has not been a diagnosis made, it could be challenging to recognize if this is a true mental health crisis or an exacerbation of symptoms due to a physical illness. Use good judgment on the appropriate facility for transport. While this decision is outside the scope of EMS providers, Thienemann et al. recommend placement in a behavioral health unit with staff who are comfortable and familiar with medical procedures.[90]

- When assessing a child with an acute onset of behavior problems, be sure to ask the parents about any recent course of illness that could be related to strep.

- Most children with PANDAS/PANS experience separation anxiety,[91] so consider allowing the parent or other caregiver to remain with their child during transport. Separation anxiety is frightening for the child and could lead to aggressive behaviors as they attempt to get to their parents.

- Children with PANDAS/PANS who severely restrict their food and fluids intake are at significant risk for dehydration, so be prepared to assess and treat accordingly. Some children may also have a feeding tube placed, so be cautious not to dislodge it when lifting and moving the patient. Severe malnutrition can lead to dangerous cardiac problems including bradycardia, hypotension, decreased blood volume, prolonged QTc, and dysrhythmias,[92] so be sure to conduct a 12-lead EKG prior to any pharmacologic interventions.

- You may be able to address behavioral issues during transport through distraction. Ask the parents to bring a favorite toy or book, allow them to watch videos on a phone or tablet, or sing with them.

- Remember that children with PANDAS/PANS will grow up to be adults with PANDAS/PANS, needing the same type of care as children. Often, however, they are undiagnosed or underdiagnosed.

- Recognize that this can be frightening for both parents and child and work to establish trust and rapport.

Rett Syndrome

You are on scene with a 10-year-old girl who has had a seizure and has not regained consciousness. Kelly is diagnosed with Rett syndrome, is nonverbal, and has frequent seizures. Her parents administered one dose of her pre-scribed rectal diazepam. You place Kelly on the monitor, including capnog-raphy to monitor her respiratory status, and start an IV. Kelly's mother tells you that she typically has multiple seizures in a row and is concerned that she has not regained consciousness. You lift Kelly to the stretcher, lying her on her side, and prepare to manage a return of seizure activity.

Rett syndrome, first described in the literature in 1966, is a genetic disorder that occurs almost exclusively in girls but may occur very rarely in boys. The prevalence of Rett syndrome is estimated at 1 in 10,000 to 15,000 live female births worldwide.[93] Children diagnosed with Rett syndrome typically have a period of normal growth and development, followed by slowing of growth and development, and finally loss of motor functions and the acquisition of autistic-like behaviors, intellectual disabilities, and breathing difficulties.[94]

The National Institute of Neurological Disorders and Stroke (NINDS) describes four progressive stages of Rett syndrome:[95]

1. Stage 1 (Early onset)
   - Onset is between 6 and 18 months of age.
   - A subtle slowing of development occurs, which can be easily missed by parents and physicians.
   - Gross motor skills are delayed.
   - Eye contact decreases.
   - The baby may begin to lose interest in toys.

2. Stage 2 (Rapid destructive)
   - Onset between 1 and 4 years of age.
   - Purposeful use of the hands and spoken language are lost.
   - Repetitive, nonpurposeful hand movements appear (e.g., hand wringing, clapping, tapping, grasping, etc.).
   - Apnea and hyperventilation occur.
   - Autistic-like symptoms begin to appear.
   - Walking may become difficult.

3. Stage 3 (Plateau)
   - Onset between 2 and 10 years and lasts for years. Some individuals remain in this stage and do not progress to stage 4.
   - Apraxia (difficulty with the motor planning required to perform physical tasks and movements including speech) appears.
   - Autistic-like behaviors may improve.

4. Stage 4 (Late motor deterioration)
   - Mobility is limited.
   - Scoliosis may appear.
   - Muscles may become weak, spastic, or hypertonic.
   - The ability to walk may be lost.

Bone fragility

Bone mineral density, bone mineral content, and bone volume are reduced in children with Rett syndrome, which can lead to frequent fractures (up to four times more frequently than the general population) and the development of scoliosis. The fractures can lead to pain, impaired mobility, and reduced quality of life. Treatment is often surgical.[96]

Scoliosis

Scoliosis, or curvature of the spine in a C or S shape, is present in the majority of people with Rett syndrome. Its onset is typically in early childhood, as early as the first year of life, with 80% showing spine curvature by age 13. It is progressive, worsening over time. Scoliosis can cause pain and restricted mobility. Severe scoliosis can cause subsequent problems with the growth of the rib cage and compression of the spine as the curve increases, which can lead the pelvis to come into contact with the lower end of the rib cage, leading to reduced lung function and significant pain. Treatment can include bracing and surgery.[97]

Seizures

Seizures are common (60% or 80% prevalence) in individuals with Rett syndrome, with a typical onset in stage 2 or 3 around the age of 4 years and peaking in frequency between ages 7 and 12 years. Earlier onset of the symptoms and increased severity of the symptoms are correlated with a higher rate of seizure activity.[98]

Sleep disturbances

Up to 80% of people with Rett syndrome have problems with sleep, including night laughing and screaming episodes, night waking, seizures, teeth grinding, difficulty falling asleep and/or waking up. Poor sleep can lead to daytime sleepiness and an overall reduced quality of life.[99]

Communication

As the syndrome progresses, language skills are lost, although some can speak with single words or phrases. People with Rett syndrome can communicate through a variety of modalities including eye gaze, gestures, and communication boards or electronic devices. Others will laugh, cry, or scream as part of their communication. Urbanowicz et al.[100] describe a variety of communication modalities demonstrated by individuals with Rett syndrome. These include "bl[owing] raspberries" to communicate happiness and a need for attention, fidgeting to indicate discomfort, and rubbing eyes to show fatigue.[101] Individuals with Rett syndrome are generally able to choose between two items, request items or activities, request attention from others, and express happiness.[102]

Social-emotional problems

Stage 2 of the syndrome progression is associated with the onset of challenging behaviors. Behaviors exhibited during this stage include withdrawn behavior, reduced eye contact, crying, screaming, and inappropriate laughter. While these behaviors are often described as "autistic-like," parents reported in one recent study that they believed these behaviors were caused by an inability to interact or show emotions due to the physical limitations associated with Rett syndrome.[103]

Attention difficulties

Children with Rett syndrome are more inattentive and distractible when compared to typically developing children. In addition, they are slower to re-engage with a stimulus after being distracted. Children developing typically tend to improve their attention and reduce their distractibility as they age. This improvement is not seen in children with Rett syndrome.[104]

Implications for EMS

- Be prepared for seizures, either as the reason for the EMS response or as a possible occurrence during transport.
- Use caution when moving patients due to their increased risk of fractures.
- Patients may experience respiratory difficulties due to scoliosis-related issues. Be cautious when positioning the patient on the stretcher or stair chair.
- Patients may have better *receptive language* (understanding) than *expressive language* (speaking). Patients may have a variety of ways to communicate. Be sure to work with the family or other caregivers to help determine what they are trying to communicate to you and to better understand their answers to your questions.
- Consider giving them a choice of answers when asking assessment questions ("Do you have a headache or a stomachache?") and use pictures if appropriate.
- Bring mobility and communication devices with you during transport.

Sickle Cell Disease

You are dispatched to a local elementary school for a nine-year-old girl with an altered mental status. Upon your arrival, you are directed to the nurse's office. Your patient, Megan, is lying on the bed, eyes open, looking unwell. The nurse tells you that Megan has a diagnosis of sickle cell disease. She recently experienced a vaso-occlusive crisis and returned to school a few days ago. Her classroom teacher alerted the nurse when Megan became weak and had difficulty holding her pencil. When you ask Megan if she has any pain, she says she has a headache, but her speech is slightly hard to understand, and she appears somewhat confused. Her blood sugar is normal. Because you are aware of the increased risk for strokes in people with sickle cell disease, even in children, you complete a stroke scale and find that Megan is positive for arm drift and unclear speech. The nurse says that Megan's dad will be meeting you at the emergency department, and the assistant principal will ride with you in the passenger seat of the ambulance.

Sickle cell disease is a genetic disorder related to a mutation in chromosome 11. It causes abnormalities in the structure of red blood cells, which function to carry oxygen-rich hemoglobin throughout the body. When a person has sickle cell disease, their red blood cells are not round discs but are elongated and curved into a crescent or sickle shape (fig. 8–1).

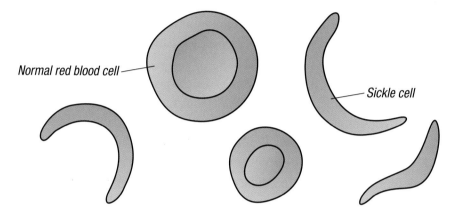

Fig. 8–1. Red blood cells are elongated and curved in people with sickle cell disease.

When red blood cells are not in the typical round shape, they are not as flexible and cannot travel through blood vessels as easily, often sticking to the blood vessel walls. When this happens, oxygen does not get to the body's tissues, causing severe pain and organ damage.

Additionally, sickled red blood cells do not live as long as normal red blood cells. Normal red blood cells live three to four months, whereas sickled red blood cells live less than three weeks. The body is often unable to keep up with the fast-paced need for new blood cells, causing the person to have anemia.

Sickle cell disease is found primarily in people of African and Afro-Caribbean descent. According to the Centers for Disease Control and Prevention, there are approximately 100,000 Americans living with sickle cell disease.[105] It occurs in about 1 in 365 Black/African-American births[106] and 1 in 16,300 Hispanic-American births.

Because sickle cell disease is a genetic condition, it is present at birth, and signs and symptoms can manifest in the first year of life. Children and adults with sickle cell disease have frequent visits to the emergency department to manage symptoms associated with the disease, many of which result in hospital admission.[107] Sickle cell disease is associated with sudden death in adults, with a median age of death of 40 years.[108] Although the cause of death is sometimes unclear, most of the deaths are attributed to cardiac or pulmonary issues.[109]

What is a sickle cell crisis?

A vaso-occlusive crisis, or *sickle cell crisis*, occurs when the red blood cells get stuck in blood vessels causing pain (often severe), tissue ischemia, and damage to joints and organs.[110] Pain accompanying a vaso-occlusive crisis can occur anywhere in the body but is most often found in the arms, legs, back, chest, and abdomen. It is typically bilateral, symmetrical, and in more than one site.[111]

A vaso-occlusive crisis can be triggered by a variety of factors including infection, illness, dehydration, physical exertion, stress, alcohol, pregnancy, and hot/cold temperatures.[112]

A vaso-occlusive crisis can contribute to a variety of complications in addition to pain, discussed in more detail below.

Signs/Symptoms of Sickle Cell Disease That May Contribute to an EMS Response

Pain and pain management

When the sickle-shaped blood cells get stuck in blood vessels, the decreased blood flow and subsequent decrease in oxygen to body tissues can cause acute, severe pain anywhere in the body. People with sickle cell disease often live with chronic pain due to long-term damage to the body.[113]

Inoue et al. report that pain management is often delayed for a variety of reasons, including emergency department wait times and the need for laboratory tests.[114] Their research also found that female patients often had a longer time to achieve pain management than did male patients, even though women tended to report greater pain.[115] This delay in pain management in the hospital setting may lead people to call 911 for pain relief.

Because of the chronic nature of their pain, patients with sickle cell disease may cope with pain in ways that are unexpected. Matthie and Jenerette[116] describe some coping strategies of people with sickle cell disease as "passive,"[117] meaning they may ignore the pain or cope through prayer or meditation. Others may take more active coping strategies, seeking distraction from the pain by listening to music, talking with visitors, or using their phones. Because these behaviors do not look like typical responses to pain, patients might be viewed as experiencing less pain than they report and might possibly be considered drug-seeking. As a consequence, pain relief might be withheld or reduced.

People with chronic pain can become tolerant of pain medications, needing higher or more frequent doses to obtain relief. They can develop a physical dependence, along with the risk of withdrawal if the medication is stopped abruptly. They also may develop a psychological dependence or addiction. While dependence and addiction to pain medication are valid concerns, they should not be used as reasons to deny relief to people in chronic pain.[118] Physicians are also wary of overprescribing opioids, which can possibly cause the undermanagement of pain. Inadequate pain management can cause people to appear to be drug-seeking when they ask for increased doses of pain medication.[119]

As EMS providers, our job is to alleviate suffering and withhold judgment on the possible motivations of our patients. It is important to recognize that there may be few or no objective signs of severe pain in a patient with sickle cell disease and in a sickle cell crisis. Acknowledging and believing the patient's report of pain is important and respectful of their experiences, and alleviating pain is an important aspect of prehospital care.

Anemia

Anemia occurs when a person does not have enough healthy red blood cells, which are necessary to carry oxygen via hemoglobin to the body's tissues. Because sickled red blood cells are fragile and do not live long, patients with sickle cell disease are prone to anemia. Anemia can be mild, moderate, or severe. While mild anemia can cause fatigue, more severe manifestations of anemia can cause shortness of breath, severe fatigue, dizziness, rapid or irregular heartbeats, chest pain, headache, and pallor.[120]

Enlarged spleen

Sickled red blood cells that are trapped in the spleen can cause it to enlarge and become painful. The spleen can then become damaged and weakened, putting people at increased risk of bacterial infections, including pneumonia, influenza, sepsis, meningitis, and other severe illnesses.

Acute chest syndrome

Acute chest syndrome is a common cause of death among people with sickle cell disease.[121] It is described as a "spectrum of disease"[122] that impacts the respiratory system due to decreased blood flow and oxygenation to lung tissue from sickled blood cells. Viral and bacterial infections are common, especially in children, and occur more frequently in the winter months. In addition, bone marrow necrosis can cause the release of fat emboli into the bloodstream, which can become stuck in the pulmonary blood vessels, leading to hypoxia.[123]

People with sickle cell disease are also at greater risk for *atelectasis* (complete or partial lung collapse) secondary to pulmonary infarction from decreased blood flow and from hypoventilation due to pain.[124] It may be difficult or painful to breathe deeply, especially in the presence of additional respiratory complications such as infection.

Respiratory complaints in people with sickle cell disease are similar to common respiratory complaints in those without sickle cell disease, including hypoxia, fever, tachypnea, tachycardia, wheezing, and increased work of breathing. While all patients with serious respiratory complaints should be evaluated in a clinical setting with x-rays and blood work, patients with sickle cell disease are especially at risk.

Treatment for acute chest syndrome in the prehospital setting will be similar to complaints not related to sickle cell disease:[125]

- Monitor SpO_2 and provide supplemental oxygen for patients with oxygen levels below 95%, those who complain of difficulty breathing, or those who exhibit signs of increased work of breathing.
- Consider fluid replacement for patients who are showing signs of sepsis or dehydration but be cautious about fluid overload for those who have decreased cardiac output.
- If pain is believed to be contributing to difficulty breathing or if patients are unable to breathe deeply due to pain, consider pain management, preferably nonopioid, to reduce the risk of contributing to respiratory depression.
- Consider bronchodilators for patients with wheezing or other evidence of bronchospasm (e.g., loss of plateau on waveform capnography or increased CO_2 levels).
- Consider use of corticosteroids for patients with acute symptoms.
- Consider aggressive ventilatory management (CPAP, bag valve mask, or intubation) for patients in respiratory failure.

Stroke

Patients with sickle cell disease are at increased risk for symptomatic and asymptomatic strokes, which are significant causes of death in both children and adults.[126] Oluwole et al.[127] report as many as 35% of children with sickle cell disease have asymptomatic or "silent strokes"[128] that can cause cognitive deficits and increase the risk of symptomatic strokes. This risk is more than 300 times greater than in healthy children.[129] By age 20, 11% of patients with sickle cell disease have experienced a "clinically apparent" stroke.[130]

Signs and symptoms of strokes in the sickle cell population are similar to the general population, but they may be missed in the pediatric sickle cell disease population as it is generally rare to see strokes in children.[131] Signs and symptoms include neurological deficits, aphasia, headaches, dizziness, vomiting, and vision changes.[132]

When assessing and treating patients with sickle cell disease for stroke in the prehospital setting, consider the following:[133]

- Obtain blood glucose levels and treat accordingly.
- Maintain $SpO_2 \geq 95\%$. Hypoxia can contribute to increased sickling of blood cells.
- Treat dehydration as indicated but be cautious of fluid overload to avoid pulmonary edema.
- Transport to a stroke center for possible thrombolysis if criteria are met.
- Pediatric patients should be transported to a pediatric facility.

Pulmonary hypertension

Issues with blood flow to the blood vessels in the lungs can cause vascular pressure to rise, which can lead to shortness of breath and fatigue, and is associated with an increased risk of death (as high as 50%).[134]

Cardiac damage/disease

The microscopic occlusions that occur in sickle cell disease can lead to myocardial ischemia and infarction, or a heart attack. Gladwin and Sachdev report that the coronary arteries may be unblocked but patients show abnormalities in their EKGs and elevated troponin levels that are indicative of acute myocardial infarction.[135]

Chronic anemia in sickle cell disease leads to an increase in left ventricular stroke volume with subsequent dilation of the left ventricle. Increased ventricular dilation leads to enlargement of the left ventricle or *left ventricular hypertrophy*. This leads to hypertension and cardiac damage.[136]

Patients with sickle cell disease are at risk for prolongation of the *QTc* (total length of ventricular depolarization and repolarization). A prolonged QTc (greater than 440 ms) is associated with ventricular dysrhythmias and sudden cardiac death.[137] Several common prehospital medications (including ondansetron, haloperidol, and albuterol) can prolong the QTc interval and could potentially cause a serious dysrhythmia. The CredibleMeds website (crediblemeds.org) provides a regularly updated list of medications that could cause a prolonged QTc interval.[138] CredibleMeds also has a smart phone app that can be accessed in the field. If a patient with sickle cell disease is in need of prehospital medications, conduct a 12-lead EKG to look for a prolonged QTc interval and obtain medical consultation as indicated.

Eye damage

All areas of the eye can be damaged as a result of sickle cell disease due to the vascular occlusion inherent to the disorder. Over time this can create irreversible damage to the eye and cause blindness.[139] Often the eye disease progression is asymptomatic until damage is significant.

Liver disease

Liver abnormalities are frequent in sickle cell disease. In one study, 96% of patients had some issue including abnormal liver function tests, viral hepatitis (B or C), enlarged liver, cirrhosis, and/or gallstones.[140] Some issues were directly attributed to the sickle cell disease process, while others had additional conditions (alcoholism or diabetes, for example) that may cause liver problems. But regardless of the underlying etiology, the authors attributed chronic vascular changes associated with sickle cell disease as contributing factors.

Priapism

Priapism is a persistent, often painful, erection that is common (30%–45% prevalence) in men with sickle cell disease when blood is unable to leave the penis.[141] Persistent priapism can lead to ischemia, inflammation, erectile dysfunction, and impotence.[142] Priapism lasting more than four hours is considered an emergency, with one-half of emergency department visits for priapism resulting in in-patient admission.[143]

Gallstones

Because the sickled red blood cells do not live as long as normal red blood cells, they die in greater numbers. Their destruction releases bilirubin, which can cause gallstones. Gallstones may block the common bile duct, causing severe pain. One study showed a prevalence of 25% in patients with sickle cell disease,[144] with higher incidence in the 11 to 29 years old age group. Patients with pain in the right upper quadrant should be evaluated for gallstones.

Cognitive functioning

Steen et al.[145] found that there can be "significant and substantial cognitive deficits"[146] in people with sickle cell disease that are the result of cumulative effects of the condition on the developing brain. Just as decreased blood flow to other organs can cause damage, poor blood flow and perfusion to the brain can cause diminished oxygen and glucose levels in the brain.[147] Children with sickle cell anemia had significantly lower IQs, slower processing speeds, and poorer working memories than those without.[148] These cognitive deficits increase with age. While cognitive deficits will not be the reason for an EMS call, these challenges could complicate your assessment and treatment (see chapter 3).

Mental health

Depression and anxiety are common in people with sickle cell disease due to living with chronic pain, complex medical complications, and other issues associated with living with a life-long, life-altering illness.[149]

Implications for EMS

- Be prepared to address pain, which can be severe whether it is acute or chronic.
- Treat respiratory symptoms according to presentation and local protocols.
- Monitor SpO_2 and provide supplemental oxygen as necessary. Do not give supplemental oxygen unless the patient is hypoxic or hypoxemic, as oxygen can suppress the production of red blood cells and can cause a rebound vaso-occlusive crisis when the oxygen is discontinued.[150]

- Be cautious with fluid replacement to avoid pulmonary edema as patients with sickle cell disease can also have decreased cardiac function.[151] But as dehydration can worsen a vaso-occlusive crisis, fluid replacement can be appropriate if administered carefully.[152] Oral rehydration is preferred if possible and tolerated.

- If treating pain with opioids, be especially cautious when monitoring respiratory status as people with sickle cell disease often have associated reduced lung volume.[153]

Before administering medications, conduct a 12-lead EKG to look at the patient's QTc interval to avoid administering any medications that are contraindicated for patients with a prolonged QTc and that could cause a potentially lethal dysrhythmia. As mentioned previously, CredibleMeds provides a current listing of medications that can prolong the QTc interval, available from both their website (www.CredibleMeds.org)[154] and smartphone application. Consult medical direction for additional guidance.

Systemic Lupus Erythematosus

For the second time in as many days you are heading to pick up Judy, who is 49 years old and has lupus. She is a frequent user of the 911 system. Her chief complaint is usually vague, saying she feels unwell, has pain and swelling in her joints, chest pain that upon evaluation does not have cardiac involvement, and a variety of other problems. Judy is usually friendly, but today she is grumpy, speaking abruptly to you and your crew. Once again, she is complaining of chest pain and says that her "heart is fluttering." You put her on the monitor and are surprised to see her heart rate at 144. You conduct a 12-lead ECG and see ST elevation in leads I, II, and V1–V6 with no reciprocal changes. Although you suspect pericarditis, you transmit the 12-lead ECG to medical control for guidance on hospital destination, as the closest facility is not a cardiac intervention center, and you begin to work through your chest pain/acute coronary syndrome protocols. After the call, you debrief with your crew and remind each other not to become complacent about patients you run frequently, as this time Judy was seriously ill.

Systemic lupus erythematosus, more commonly called *lupus,* is a chronic autoimmune connective tissue disease.[155] The CDC reports as many as 483,000 people are living with lupus in the United States,[156] with significantly higher rates in women and people of African descent. Lupus typically appears between the ages of 15 to 40 and has a prevalence range of 15 to 68 per 100,000.[157]

Lupus can affect multiple systems in the body, including the joints, skin, brain, lungs, kidneys, central nervous system, and cardiovascular system, causing inflammation, tissue and organ damage, and mild-to-life threatening complications. In some cases the diagnosis of lupus comes after presentation to the emergency department for worrisome cardiac, respiratory, or other symptoms (table 8–2).[158]

Table 8–2. Body systems impacted by lupus and possible symptoms or complications

Body Systems Impacted by Lupus and Possible Symptoms or Complications	
Musculoskeletal	• Pain and inflammation • Necrosis • Septic arthritis
Skin	• Rash
Brain	• Seizure • Stroke* • Altered mental status • Psychosis†
Pulmonary system	• Pulmonary hypertension • Pulmonary embolism • Respiratory infections • Diffuse alveolar hemorrhage
Cardiovascular system	• Pericarditis • Myocarditis • Endocarditis • Hypertensive crisis • Aneurysm (rare)‡

Table 8–2. ...*continued*

Renal system	• Kidney infections • Nephritis • Chronic kidney disease
Gastrointestinal system	• Pancreatitis • Acute pain • Pseudo-obstruction
Miscellaneous	• Sepsis • Headache • Mood disorders • Eye disorders (uncommon)[§]

Sources:

Marco and Chhakchhuak, "Complications of Systemic Lupus Erythematosus in the Emergency Department"; Vymetal et al., "Emergency Situations in Rheumatology with a Focus on Systemic Autoimmune Diseases"; and Pokroy-Shapira, Gelernter, and Molad, "Evolution of Chronic Kidney Disease in Patients with Systemic Lupus Erythematosus over a Long-Period Follow-up: A Single-Center Inception Cohort Study."

[*]Reshma M. Khan et al., "Embolic Stroke as the Initial Manifestation of Systemic Lupus Erythematosus."

[†] Sheena Sharma et al., "Acute Psychosis Presenting in a Patient with Systemic Lupus Erythematosus: Questions," *Pediatric Nephrology* 31, no. 2 (2015): 227–228, https://doi.org/10.1007/s00467-015-3052-3.

[‡] C. Graffeo et al., "Rapid Aneurysm Growth and Rupture in Systemic Lupus Erythematosus," *Surgical Neurology International* 6, no. 1 (2015): 9, https://doi.org/10.4103/2152-7806.149617.

[§] Man, Mok, and Fu, "Neuro-Ophthalmologic Manifestations of Systemic Lupus Erythematosus: A Systematic Review."

Cardiovascular involvement

Lupus can impact the cardiovascular system in several ways that might necessitate an EMS response.[159] Heart disease is extremely common in patients with lupus and can be exacerbated by a flare in lupus symptoms.[160] Modi et al. report as much as a 50% increase in presentations to the emergency department with chest pain in patients with lupus when compared to those without.[161] In some cases, the presentation to the emergency department with cardiac symptoms led to an initial diagnosis of lupus.[162]

Modi et al. looked at emergency department visits for 2,675 patients with lupus, with 397 having a chief complaint of chest pain and 224 subsequent hospital admissions.[163] Of those admissions, almost 43% either had discharge diagnoses of a cardiovascular complaint such as coronary artery disease, myocardial infarction, angina, or congestive heart failure, or had cardiac issues ruled out.[164] Other discharge diagnoses in the remaining 57% included costochondritis, respiratory problems such as COPD, pulmonary embolism, pneumonia, and others. The authors noted, however, that of the 173 patients who presented with chest pain who were discharged home from the emergency department, almost one-fourth did not receive a cardiac workup prior to discharge. Therefore a cardiac problem may have been missed, making the previous numbers falsely low. Despite the lack of a cardiac diagnosis in the majority of the admitted patients, the risk of cardiovascular disease in patients with lupus remains high and should always be carefully considered in the prehospital setting.

- *Pericarditis.* Pericarditis is common, and in patients with lupus, it is not related to infection. Symptoms can include substernal chest pain, tachycardia, and widespread ST elevation.[165] It can lead to cardiac tamponade.[166]

- *Valve abnormalities.* Valve abnormalities are present in as many as 60% of patients with lupus. Valve thickening or regurgitation are asymptomatic but can still lead to severe complications, including stroke, embolism, and congestive heart failure.[167]

- *Coronary artery disease.* Coronary artery disease is very common in patients with lupus (as much as 10 times higher compared to the general population) and must be considered in all patients, even young adults, with chest pain or other symptoms.[168] Do not neglect to conduct an EKG in patients with lupus and chest pain, even if they do not fit the typical presentation of a patient with coronary artery disease or do not have increased risk factors typical of coronary artery disease (age, gender, family history, etc.).

Pulmonary involvement

- *Pulmonary arterial hypertension.* Pulmonary arterial hypertension occurs when there is high blood pressure in the pulmonary artery (the vessel that takes blood from the heart back to the lungs) due to narrowing or blockage. Because of the increased work of the heart needed to pump blood through the narrow vessels, cardiac muscle weakness and right-sided heart failure can occur.[169]

Pulmonary arterial hypertension is a life-threatening complication of lupus, occurring in as many as 14% of patients.[170] The mortality rate is as high as 50% in emergency situations, and death within 24 hours of admission to the emergency department is common.

The workup for a diagnosis of pulmonary arterial hypertension includes an EKG and a right heart catheterization to look at pressure within the artery.[171] Treatment in the field should include an EKG, monitoring and managing the patient's vital signs and hemodynamic stability, and management of symptoms according to your local protocols or medical direction.

- *Pleuritis.* Also known as *pleurisy*, pleuritis is an inflammation of lung tissues and is the most common respiratory complication of lupus.[172] Its symptoms include pain, shortness of breath, and shallow breathing or other difficulty with breathing. Because lupus has so many significant cardiac complications, it is important not to misinterpret cardiac pain for pleuritic pain.[173]

- *Shrinking lung syndrome.* This syndrome is caused by dysfunction of the diaphragm, which leads to restriction of the lungs and subsequent difficulty breathing and pain.[174]

- *Pulmonary embolism.* People with lupus are at an increased risk of pulmonary embolism, which should be considered if patients present with a sudden onset of hypoxia and difficulty breathing coupled with tachycardia and chest pain.[175]

- *Pneumonia and acute lupus pneumonitis.* Pneumonia (associated with infection) and acute lupus pneumonitis (associated with a lupus flare) can be an emergency. It is difficult to differentiate between them as the symptoms of difficulty breathing, hypoxia, cough, fever, and positive chest x-ray are similar in both conditions. The mortality rate of acute lupus pneumonitis is high (50%).[176]

- *Diffuse alveolar hemorrhage.* Diffuse alveolar hemorrhage refers to bleeding from the lung tissue, and it is a rare but life-threatening condition, with death rates as high as 50% to 90%. Symptoms include difficulty breathing, hypoxia, tachypnea, tachycardia, and *hemoptysis* (bloody sputum).[177]

Many of these pulmonary complications cannot be effectively treated in the prehospital setting except for symptom management. As per your local protocols, provide supplementary oxygen as appropriate, and bronchodilators and CPAP as indicated.

Renal involvement

- *Lupus nephritis.* Lupus nephritis, or inflammation of the kidneys, occurs in as many as 50% to 70% of people with lupus.[178] Symptoms include edema, hypertension, and dark urine. If lupus nephritis is not treated or well-controlled, it can lead to renal failure and death.[179]

- *Chronic kidney disease.* Chronic kidney disease is a common complication of lupus that can lead to hypertension and edema in the arms and legs.[180] In addition, chronic kidney disease can also contribute to cardiovascular disease with heart disease worsening as the kidney disease progresses.[181]

Musculoskeletal involvement

More than 90% of people with lupus have problems with bones and joints.[182] Joint pain, inflammation, and deformity primarily occur in the feet, wrists, and hands and may be the first symptoms to appear at the onset of the disease process.[183]

Avascular bone necrosis/osteonecrosis

Another serious complication is *bone necrosis* (bone death), which can happen when the blood supply to the bones is reduced or interrupted. It is also linked to steroid use (common in treating other symptoms of lupus) and alcohol use.[184] Symptomatic bone necrosis occurs in upwards of 15% of people with lupus but may be as high as 40% in patients without symptoms.[185]

The early course of bone necrosis can be asymptomatic. The symptoms start with pain in the bone when pressure is applied. As the disease progresses, the pain can become constant and more severe. The disease can eventually lead to collapse of the bone and nearby joints.[186] The most commonly affected joints are the hips and knees, but it can occur in any joint.[187] A study conducted by Gladman et al.[188] reported an average onset of bone necrosis at approximately eight years post diagnosis, and almost half of the participants in the study had multiple joint involvement at the initial necrosis diagnosis. Surgery and reducing steroid use are common interventions.

Gastrointestinal involvement

Gastrointestinal involvement may involve the following:

- *Pseudo-obstruction.* A pseudo-obstruction occurs when there are symptoms of a bowel obstruction (pain, nausea, vomiting, constipation, and abdominal distention) but no actual obstruction.[189]
- *Acute abdominal pain.* This pain can be related to lupus (mesenteric vasculitis or pancreatitis) or not related (appendicitis, gallbladder disease/inflammation, ulcers, etc.).[190]

Prehospital interventions for gastrointestinal complications associated with lupus include pain management and monitoring vital signs for hemodynamic stability.

Sepsis

Infections are a common consequence of the inherent immunosuppression that is characteristic of lupus, as well as a consequence of the common therapeutic treatments for lupus. Patients with lupus are frequently treated with steroids, immunosuppressives, and other medications that allow for opportunistic infections to flourish.[191] Patients with lupus can be more severely affected by these infections, which can lead to sepsis, septic shock, and death. Barrett et al. report that as many as 50% of patients with lupus will experience at least one severe infection in their lives.[192] It is also a significant contributor to deaths associated with lupus.[193]

Stroke

Antiphospholipid syndrome, which causes thromboses to occur, is associated with lupus and can potentially lead to deep vein thrombosis, pulmonary embolism, myocardial infarction, and pulmonary hypertension.[194] This syndrome can also lead to an increased risk (up to 20%) of cerebrovascular events, including transient ischemic attacks, ischemic strokes, and hemorrhagic strokes.[195] Strokes contribute up to an estimated 20% to 30% of deaths in people with lupus.[196]

Eye disorders

While problems with the eyes or vision are a less common manifestation of lupus, they can cause significant disability and impair quality of life.[197]

- Optic neuropathy can cause eye pain, decreased acuity (vision loss) and partial loss of vision (blind spots). It can be effectively treated with corticosteroids.

- Visual field defects whereby the total area of vision is reduced can be caused by problems with the eye vasculature.

- Patients with lupus and myasthenia gravis can have eyelid drooping and eye muscle weakness or paralysis.

Mood disorders

Lupus is a difficult disease to manage and live with, causing widespread pain and fatigue. It is a life-long disease with complex body system involvement, no cure, and complicated treatments. Not surprisingly, it is common (in as many as 75% of people) for lupus to contribute to the development of a mood disorder.[198] Researchers have considered that there is a correlation between the presence of an autoimmune disorder and mood disorders.[199] Varying types of mood disorders are present with patients with lupus and can contribute to a lower quality of life.[200]

- *Anxiety and depression.* Anxiety and depression are common in patients with lupus and can be correlated to living with chronic pain, especially with more severe pain.[201] The presence of anxiety and depression in patients with lupus varies by study but has been reported as high as 47% (any mood or anxiety disorder) compared to 17% in the general population. Major depression is reported at 22% and 5%, respectively, and anxiety disorders reported at almost 29% and 12%, respectively.[202] Alsowaida et al. reported a high incidence (62%) of noncompliance with taking prescribed medications for depression and suggest that increased disease activity/symptoms contribute to the severity of depression symptoms.[203]

- *Alexithymia.* Alexithymia is a mood disorder characterized by difficulty recognizing and identifying one's own emotional states. It can manifest with poor emotional awareness and difficulties with social and personal relationships, and it can lead to diminished capability to respond well to stress.[204] Alexithymia is estimated to occur in as many as 61% of people with lupus.[205]

Pregnancy complications

Because lupus is primarily diagnosed in women of childbearing age, concerns surrounding pregnancy are important to consider. Buyon et al. reported that 81% of patients with stable and mild/moderate lupus had uncomplicated pregnancies,[206] but the complications that do arise can be severe. Some complications associated with lupus and pregnancy include fetal death, placental insufficiency, small-for-gestational-age babies, hypertension, premature birth, and preeclampsia. An increased risk for premature birth and preeclampsia are found also in pregnant women with lupus and a history of nephritis.

Other associated conditions

Other conditions associated with lupus include headache and seizures.[207]

Childhood-onset lupus

For children, the onset of symptoms may be similar to the adult onset of the disease, but the onset is generally more severe. In one-third of pediatric cases, lupus can have an atypical presentation that can delay or complicate diagnosis and intervention.[208]

- *Pulmonary complications.* Pulmonary complications are reported to be the same or less frequent in children versus adults, with the most frequent problems reported being pleuritis, pneumonia, chronic lung disease, pulmonary hypertension, and pulmonary hemorrhage.

- *Gastrointestinal symptoms.* Gastrointestinal symptoms are common and can be severe in children. The most common cause is due to mesenteric vasculitis, which can cause nausea, vomiting, diarrhea, bloating, and pain/tenderness, and it may lead to necrosis or bowel perforation. Other rare complications include pancreatitis, peritonitis, and pseudo-obstruction.

- *Cardiac signs.* Cardiac signs of childhood-onset lupus are most commonly manifested as pericarditis, myocarditis, and endocarditis. Valve problems and coronary artery disease are less common when compared to the adult onset course of the disease. Myocardial infarction is rare in children with lupus, but childhood onset of lupus is a risk factor for early atherosclerosis and subsequent cardiovascular disease.

Implications for EMS

- Patients with lupus are at risk for frequent use of the emergency department,[209] so you may see some patients frequently. Do not neglect to conduct a thorough assessment, as a new or infrequent onset of symptoms can be life-threatening.

- Take all reports of chest pain seriously. Conduct a thorough assessment, including a 12-lead EKG, on all patients with chest pain or other potential cardiac symptoms, even if they do not meet the classic demographics for coronary artery disease.

- Be prepared to manage symptoms as they present in accordance with your local protocols.

- Patients with lupus live with chronic and often severe pain, which can contribute to depression and anxiety.

- Consider sepsis for patients who meet physiological criteria due to increased risk factors and infectious opportunity.

Notes

1. US Department of Health and Human Services, Center for Behavioral Health Statistics and Quality, *Behavioral Health Trends in the United States: Results from the 2014 National Survey on Drug Use and Health*, HHS Publication No. SMA 15-4927, NSDUH Series H-50 (Rockville, MD: US Dept. of HHS, Substance Abuse and Mental Health Services Administration, CBHSQ, 2015), retrieved from http://www.samhsa.gov/data/.

2. Tom Parkman et al., "Qualitative Exploration of Why People Repeatedly Attend Emergency Departments for Alcohol-Related Reasons," *Bio Med Central Health Services Research* 17 (2017): 1–9, https://doi.org/10.1186/s12913-017-2091-9.

3. Tom Parkman et al., "Qualitative Exploration of Why People Repeatedly Attend Emergency Departments for Alcohol-Related Reasons,"

4. US Department of Health and Human Services, Center for Behavioral Health Statistics and Quality, "Behavioral Health Trends in the United States: Results from the 2014 National Survey on Drug Use and Health."

5. US Department of Health and Human Services, Center for Behavioral Health Statistics and Quality, "Behavioral Health Trends in the United States: Results from the 2014 National Survey on Drug Use and Health," 19.

6. US Department of Health and Human Services, Center for Behavioral Health Statistics and Quality, "Behavioral Health Trends in the United States: Results from the 2014 National Survey on Drug Use and Health," 19.

7. US Department of Health and Human Services, Center for Behavioral Health Statistics and Quality, "Behavioral Health Trends in the United States: Results from the 2014 National Survey on Drug Use and Health."

8. American Psychiatric Association, *Diagnostic and Statistical Manual of Mental Disorders*, 4th ed. (Washington, DC: APA, 1994).

9. American Psychiatric Association, *Diagnostic and Statistical Manual of Mental Disorders*, 5th ed. (Washington, DC: APA, 2013).

10. American Psychiatric Association, *Diagnostic and Statistical Manual of Mental Disorders*, 5th ed., 490–491.

11. Michaël Schwarzinger et al., "Alcohol Use Disorders and Associated Chronic Disease—A National Retrospective Cohort Study from France," *BioMed Central Public Health* 18, no. 1 (2018): 1–9, https://doi.org/10.1186/s12889-017-4587-y.

12. Marissa B. Esser et al., "Prevalence of Alcohol Dependence among US Adult Drinkers, 2009–2011," *Preventing Chronic Disease* 11 (2014): 1–11, https://doi.org/10.5888/pcd11.140329.

13. Schwarzinger et al., "Alcohol Use Disorders and Associated Chronic Disease."

14. Maurizio Baldassarre et al., "Accesses for Alcohol Intoxication to the Emergency Department and the Risk of Re-hospitalization: An Observational Retrospective Study," *Addictive Behaviors* 77 (2018): 1–6, https://doi.org/10.1016/j.addbeh.2017.08.031.

15. US Department of Health and Human Services, Centers for Disease Control and Prevention, "Alcohol and Public Health: Alcohol-Related Disease Impact (ARDI)," 2013, retrieved March 11, 2018, https://nccd.cdc.gov/dph_ardi/.

16. Kevin D. Shield, Charles Parry, and Jurgen Rehm, "Chronic Diseases and Conditions Related to Alcohol Use," *Alcohol Research: Current Reviews* 35, no. 2 (2013): 155–172, retrieved March 17, 2018, https://www.ncbi.nlm.nih.gov/pmc/articles/PMC3908707/; and Matti Hillbom, Ilkka Pieninkeroinen, and Maurizio Leone, "Seizures in Alcohol Dependent Patients: Epidemiology, Pathophysiology, and Management," *CNS Drugs* 17, no. 14 (2003): 1,013–1,030, https://doi.org/10.2165/00023210-200317140-00002.

17. Baldassarre et al., "Accesses for Alcohol Intoxication to the Emergency Department and the Risk of Re-hospitalization."

18. J. Kornusky and G. Cabrera, *Alcohol Withdrawal Syndrome: Delirium Tremens* (Glendale, CA: Cinahl Information Systems, 2018).

19. Stefano Gitto et al., "Multidisciplinary View of Alcohol Use Disorder: From a Psychiatric Illness to a Major Liver Disease," *Biomolecules* 6, no. 1 (2016): 1–12, https://doi.org/10.3390/biom6010011.

20. Schwarzinger et al., "Alcohol Use Disorders and Associated Chronic Disease."

21. Gitto et al., "Multidisciplinary View of Alcohol Use Disorder."

22. Gitto et al., "Multidisciplinary View of Alcohol Use Disorder"; and US Department of Health and Human Services, National Institutes of Health, National Cancer Institute, "Alcohol and Cancer Risk," June 24, 2013, retrieved July 3, 2018, https://www.cancer.gov/about-cancer/causes-prevention/risk/alcohol/alcohol-fact-sheet.

23. Gitto et al., "Multidisciplinary View of Alcohol Use Disorder"; A. Mahli and C. Hellerbrand, "Alcohol and Obesity: A Dangerous Association for Fatty Liver Disease," *Digestive Diseases* 34, Supplement 1 (2016): 32–39, https://doi.org/10.1159/000447279.

24. A. Desai, H. Panchal, and H. Parmar, "Acute Pancreatitis: Causes, Pathophysiology, Different Modalities of Management," *International Archives of Integrated Medicine* 13, no. 4 (2016): 66–71.

25. US Department of Health and Human Services, National Institutes of Health, National Institute of Diabetes and Digestive and Kidney Diseases, "Pancreatitis," November 1, 2017, retrieved March 17, 2018, https://www.niddk.nih.gov/health-information/digestive-diseases/pancreatitis/all-content.

26. Mats Ramstedt, "Alcohol and Pancreatitis Mortality at the Population Level: Experiences from 14 Western Countries," *Addiction* 99, no. 10 (2004): 1,255–1,261, https://doi.org/10.1111/j.1360-0443.2004.00798.x.

27. Hillbom, Pieninkeroinen, and Leone, "Seizures in Alcohol Dependent Patients: Epidemiology, Pathophysiology, and Management."

28. Hillbom, Pieninkeroinen, and Leone, "Seizures in Alcohol Dependent Patients: Epidemiology, Pathophysiology, and Management."

29. Raihan Khalid and Marijane Leonard, "Bleeding Esophageal Varices: Overview, Causes, and Risk Factors," April 20, 2017, retrieved March 17, 2018, https://www.healthline.com/health/bleeding-esophageal-varices.

30. Tsung-Hsing Hung et al., "A Fourfold Increase of Oesophageal Variceal Bleeding in Cirrhotic Patients with a History of Oesophageal Variceal Bleeding," *Singapore Medical Journal* 57, no. 9 (2016): 511–513, https://doi.org/10.11622/smedj.2015177.

31. Jussi M. Kärkkäinen et al., "Alcohol Abuse Increases Rebleeding Risk and Mortality on Patients with Non-Variceal Upper Gastrointestinal Bleeding," *Digestive Diseases and Sciences* 60, no. 12 (2015): 3,707–3,715, https://doi.org/10.1007/s10620-015-3806-6.

32. Philip N. Salen, "Wernicke Encephalopathy," January 7, 2017, retrieved March 17, 2018, https://emedicine.medscape.com/article/794583-overview.

33. Salen, "Wernicke Encephalopathy."

34. Salen, "Wernicke Encephalopathy."

35. Salen, "Wernicke Encephalopathy."

36. Herbert L. Muncie, Jr., Yasmin Yasinian, and Linda Oge, "Outpatient Management of Alcohol Withdrawal Syndrome," *American Family Physician* 88, no. 9 (2013): 589–595, retrieved from http://www.aafp.org/afp; and Hillbom, Pieninkeroinen, and Leone, "Seizures in Alcohol Dependent Patients: Epidemiology, Pathophysiology, and Management."

37. Muncie, Yasinian, and Oge, "Outpatient Management of Alcohol Withdrawal Syndrome."

38. Muncie, Yasinian, and Oge, "Outpatient Management of Alcohol Withdrawal Syndrome."

39. Muncie, Yasinian, and Oge, "Outpatient Management of Alcohol Withdrawal Syndrome."

40. Ulf Berggren et al., "Thrombocytopenia in Early Alcohol Withdrawal Is Associated with Development of Delirium Tremens or Seizures," *Alcohol and Alcoholism* 44, no. 4 (2009): 382–386, https://doi.org/10.1093/alcalc/agp012.

41. Berggren et al., "Thrombocytopenia in Early Alcohol Withdrawal Is Associated with Development of Delirium Tremens or Seizures"; and Hillbom, Pieninkeroinen, and Leone, "Seizures in Alcohol Dependent Patients: Epidemiology, Pathophysiology, and Management."

42. Hillbom, Pieninkeroinen, and Leone, "Seizures in Alcohol Dependent Patients: Epidemiology, Pathophysiology, and Management."

43. Hillbom, Pieninkeroinen, and Leone, "Seizures in Alcohol Dependent Patients: Epidemiology, Pathophysiology, and Management."

44. Muncie, Yasinian, and Oge, "Outpatient Management of Alcohol Withdrawal Syndrome."

45. Brian K. Walsh, Michael P. Czervinske, and Robert M. DiBlasi, *Neonatal and Pediatric Respiratory Care* (St. Louis, MO: Elsevier, 2010).

46. Cystic Fibrosis Foundation, *Cystic Fibrosis Foundation Patient Registry 2014 Annual Data Report* (Bethesda, MD: Cystic Fibrosis Foundation, 2015), 10, https://www.cff.org/2014-Annual-Data-Report.pdf.

47. Cystic Fibrosis Foundation, *Cystic Fibrosis Foundation Patient Registry 2014 Annual Data Report*.

48. Cystic Fibrosis Foundation, "About Cystic Fibrosis: What is CF?" retrieved November 19, 2017, https://www.cff.org/What-is-CF/About-Cystic-Fibrosis/.

49. S. Naehrig, C. M. Chao, and L. Naehrlich, "Cystic Fibrosis: Diagnosis and Treatment," *Deutsches Aerzteblatt International* 114 (2017): 564-574, https://doi.org/10.3238/arztebl.2017.0564.

50. Cystic Fibrosis Foundation, *Cystic Fibrosis Foundation Patient Registry 2014 Annual Data Report*; and L. Oud, "Critical Illness among Adults with Cystic Fibrosis in Texas, 2004–2013: Patterns of ICU Utilization, Characteristics, and Outcomes," *PLoS ONE* 12, no. 10 (2017): 1–17, https://doi.org/10.1371/journal.pone.0186770.

51. Oud, "Critical Illness among Adults with Cystic Fibrosis in Texas, 2004–2013."

52. Atul Gupta, Donald Urquhart, and Mark Rosenthal, "Marked Improvement in Cystic Fibrosis Lung Disease and Nutrition following Change in Home Environment," *Journal of the Royal Society of Medicine* 102, 1 (supp.) (2009): 45–48, https://doi.org/10.1258/jrsm.2009.s19010.

53. Naehrig, Chao, and Naehrlich, "Cystic Fibrosis: Diagnosis and Treatment"; Walsh, Czervinske, and DiBlasi, *Neonatal and Pediatric Respiratory Care*.

54. Sarath C. Ranganathan et al., "Early Lung Disease in Infants and Preschool Children with Cystic Fibrosis: What Have We Learned and What Should We Do about It?" *American Journal of Respiratory and Critical Care Medicine* 195, no. 12 (2017): 1,567–1,575, https://doi.org/10.1164/rccm.201606-1107ci.

55. US Department of Health and Human Services, National Institutes of Health, National Heart, Lung, and Blood Institute, "What Is Bronchiectasis?" June 2, 2014, retrieved November 24, 2017, https://www.nhlbi.nih.gov/health/health-topics/topics/brn.

56. Naehrig, Chao, and Naehrlich, "Cystic Fibrosis: Diagnosis and Treatment."

57. Atqah AbdulWahab et al., "The Emergence of Multidrug-Resistant Pseudomonas Aeruginosa in Cystic Fibrosis Patients on Inhaled Antibiotics," *Lung India* 34, no. 6 (2017): 527–531, https://doi.org/10.4103/lungindia.lungindia_39_17.

58. Naehrig, Chao, Naehrlich, "Cystic Fibrosis: Diagnosis and Treatment"; Markus Wettstein, Lorenz Radlinger, Thomas Riedel, "Effect of Different Breathing Aids on Ventilation Distribution in Adults with Cystic Fibrosis," *PLoS ONE* 9, no. 9 (2014): 1–5, https://doi.org/10.1371/journal.pone.0106591; Adriana Haack and Maria R. Garbi Novaes, "Multidisciplinary Care in Cystic Fibrosis: A Clinical-Nutrition Review," *Nutrición Hospitalaria* 27, no. 2 (2012): 362–371, https://www.ncbi.nlm.nih.gov/pubmed/22732957; and Walsh, Czervinske, and DiBlasi, *Neonatal and Pediatric Respiratory Care*.

59. Courtney M. Wheatley et al., "Effects of Exercise Intensity Compared to Albuterol in Individuals with Cystic Fibrosis," *Respiratory Medicine* 109, no. 4 (2015): 463–474, https://doi.org/10.1016/j.rmed.2014.12.002.

60. Connor Lewis et al., "Diabetes-Related Mortality in Adults with Cystic Fibrosis: Role of Genotype and Sex," *American Journal of Respiratory and Critical Care Medicine* 191, no. 2 (2015), 194–200, https://doi.org/10.1164/rccm.201403-0576oc.

61. Lewis et al., "Diabetes-Related Mortality in Adults with Cystic Fibrosis: Role of Genotype and Sex."

62. Katja Konrad et al., "Cystic Fibrosis-Related Diabetes Compared to Type 1 and Type 2 Diabetes in Adults," *Diabetes/Metabolism Research and Reviews* 29, no. 7 (2013): 568–575, https://doi.org/10.1002/dmrr.2429.

63. Donal O'Shea and Jean O'Connell, "Cystic Fibrosis Related Diabetes," *Current Diabetes Reports* 14, no. 511 (2014): 1–10, https://doi.org/10.1007/s11892-014-0511-3.

64. Konrad et al., "Cystic Fibrosis-Related Diabetes Compared to Type 1 and Type 2 Diabetes in Adults."

65. Harold Tabori et al., "Abdominal Symptoms in Cystic Fibrosis and Their Relation to Genotype, History, Clinical and Laboratory Findings," *PLoS ONE* 12, no. 5 (2017): 1–19, https://doi.org/10.1371/journal.pone.0174463.

66. Hasan M. Isa, Lina F. Al-Ali, and Afaf M. Mohamed, "Growth Assessment and Risk Factors of Malnutrition in Children with Cystic Fibrosis," *Saudi Medical Journal* 37, no. 3 (2016): 293–298, https://doi.org/10.15537/smj.2016.3.13476.

67. Walsh, Czervinske, and DiBlasi, *Neonatal and Pediatric Respiratory Care.*

68. R. Hankard, A. Munck, and J. Navarro, "Nutrition and Growth in Cystic Fibrosis," *Hormone Research in Paediatrics* 58, no. S1 (2002): 16–20, https://doi.org/10.1159/000064763.

69. Isa, Al-Ali, and Mohamed, "Growth Assessment and Risk Factors of Malnutrition in Children with Cystic Fibrosis"; and R. Hankard, A. Munck, and J. Navarro, "Nutrition and Growth in Cystic Fibrosis."

70. Isa, Al-Ali, and Mohamed, "Growth Assessment and Risk Factors of Malnutrition in Children with Cystic Fibrosis."

71. Lisa J. Meltzer and Suzanne E. Beck, "Sleep Patterns in Children with Cystic Fibrosis," *Children's Health Care* 41, no. 3 (2012): 260–268, https://doi.org/10.1080/02739615.2012.686365.

72. Ian Ketchell, "Patients with Cystic Fibrosis Should Be Intubated and Ventilated," *Journal of the Royal Society of Medicine* 103, no. S1 (2010): 20–24, https://doi.org/10.1258/jrsm.2010.s11005.

73. US Department of Health and Human Services, National Institutes of Health, National Institute of Mental Health, Office of Science Policy, Planning, and Communications, Science Writing, Press, and Dissemination Branch, *PANDAS—Questions and Answers*, Publication No. OM 16-4309 (Bethesda, MD: NIH, NIMH, 2016), https://www.nimh.nih.gov/health/publications/pandas/pandas-qa-508_01272017_154202.pdf.

74. Susan E. Swedo, Jennifer Frankovich, and Tanya K. Murphy, "Overview of Treatment of Pediatric Acute-Onset Neuropsychiatric Syndrome," *Journal of Child and Adolescent Psychopharmacology* 27, no. 7 (2017): 562–565, https://doi.org/10.1089/cap.2017.0042.

75. Lisa A. Snider and Susan E. Swedo, "PANDAS: Current Status and Directions for Research," *Molecular Psychiatry* 9, no. 10 (2004): 900–907, https://doi.org/10.1038/sj.mp.4001542.

76. Swedo, Frankovich, and Murphy, "Overview of Treatment of Pediatric Acute-Onset Neuropsychiatric Syndrome."

77. US Department of HHS, NIH, NIMH, *PANDAS—Questions and Answers.*

78. Margo Thienemann et al., "Clinical Management of Pediatric Acute-Onset Neuropsychiatric Syndrome: Part I–Psychiatric and Behavioral Interventions," *Journal of Child and Adolescent Psychopharmacology* 27, no. 7 (2017): 1–8, https://doi.org/10.1089/cap.2016.0145; Tanya K. Murphy, Diana M. Gerardi, and E. Carla Parker-Athill, "The PANDAS Controversy: Why (and How) Is It Still Unsettled?" *Current Developmental Disorders Reports* 1, no. 4 (2014): 236–244, https://doi.org/10.1007/s40474-014-0025-3; and Daniel Demesh, Jordan M. Virbalas, and John P. Bent, "The Role of Tonsillectomy in the Treatment of Pediatric Autoimmune Neuropsychiatric Disorders Associated with Streptococcal Infections (PANDAS)," *JAMA Otolaryngology–Head & Neck Surgery* 141, no. 3 (2015): 272–275, https://doi.org/10.1001/jamaoto.2014.3407.

79. Thienemann et al., "Clinical Management of Pediatric Acute-Onset Neuropsychiatric Syndrome: Part I," 1.

80. S. Esposito et al., "Pediatric Autoimmune Neuropsychiatric Disorders Associated with Streptococcal Infections: An Overview," *European Journal of Clinical Microbiology & Infectious Diseases* 33, no. 12 (2014): 2,105–2,109, https://doi.org/10.1007/s10096-014-2185-9; and US Department of HHS, NIH, NIMH, *PANDAS—Questions and Answers.*

81. Michael S. Cooperstock et al., "Clinical Management of Pediatric Acute-Onset Neuropsychiatric Syndrome: Part III—Treatment and Prevention of Infections," *Journal of Child and Adolescent Psychopharmacology* 27, no. 7 (2017): 1–13, https://doi.org/10.1089/cap.2016.0151; and Murphy, Gerardi, and Parker-Athill, "The PANDAS Controversy: Why (and How) Is It Still Unsettled?"

82. Murphy, Gerardi, and Parker-Athill, "The PANDAS Controversy: Why (and How) Is It Still Unsettled?"; and Suhas Doshi, Rajeesh Maniar, and Girish Banwari, "Pediatric Autoimmune Neuropsychiatric Disorders Associated with Streptococcal Infections (PANDAS)," *Indian Journal of Pediatrics* 82, no. 5 (2014): 480–481, https://doi.org/10.1007/s12098-014-1641-y.

83. Sonja Orlovska et al., "Association of Streptococcal Throat Infection with Mental Disorders," *JAMA Psychiatry* 74, no. 7 (2017): 740, https://doi.org/10.1001/jamapsychiatry.2017.0995.

84. Thienemann et al., "Clinical Management of Pediatric Acute-Onset Neuropsychiatric Syndrome: Part I."

85. Swedo, Frankovich, and Murphy, "Overview of Treatment of Pediatric Acute-Onset Neuropsychiatric Syndrome."

86. Cooperstock et al., "Clinical Management of Pediatric Acute-Onset Neuropsychiatric Syndrome: Part III—Treatment and Prevention of Infections"; Jennifer Frankovich et al., "Clinical Management of Pediatric Acute-Onset Neuropsychiatric Syndrome: Part II—Use of Immunomodulatory Therapies," *Journal of Child and Adolescent Psychopharmacology* 27, no. 7 (2017), 1–16, https://doi.org/10.1089/cap.2016.0148.

87. Thienemann et al., "Clinical Management of Pediatric Acute-Onset Neuropsychiatric Syndrome: Part I"; Swedo, Frankovich, and Murphy, "Overview of Treatment of Pediatric Acute-Onset Neuropsychiatric Syndrome"; J. Tan, C. Smith, and R. Goldman, "Pediatric Autoimmune Neuropsychiatric Disorders Associated with Streptococcal Infections," *Canadian Family Physician* 58 (2012): 957–959; S. Esposito et al., "Pediatric Autoimmune Neuropsychiatric Disorders Associated with Streptococcal Infections: An Overview"; and Demesh, Virbalas, and Bent, "The Role of Tonsillectomy in the Treatment of Pediatric Autoimmune Neuropsychiatric Disorders Associated with Streptococcal Infections (PANDAS)."

88. Thienemann et al., "Clinical Management of Pediatric Acute-Onset Neuropsychiatric Syndrome: Part I."

89. Thienemann et al., "Clinical Management of Pediatric Acute-Onset Neuropsychiatric Syndrome: Part I."

90. Thienemann et al., "Clinical Management of Pediatric Acute-Onset Neuropsychiatric Syndrome: Part I."

91. Thienemann et al., "Clinical Management of Pediatric Acute-Onset Neuropsychiatric Syndrome: Part I."

92. J. G. Webb, M. C. Kiess, and C. C. Chan-Yan, "Malnutrition and the Heart," *Canadian Medical Association Journal* 135, no. 7 (1986): 753–758.

93. US Department of Health and Human Services, National Institutes of Health, National Institute of Neurological Disorders and Stroke, "Rett Syndrome," May 9, 2017, retrieved May 21, 2018, https://www.ninds.nih.gov/Disorders/Patient-Caregiver-Education/Fact-Sheets/Rett-Syndrome-Fact-Sheet.

94. US Department of Health and Human Services, NIH, NINDS, "Rett Syndrome."

95. US Department of Health and Human Services, NIH, NINDS, "Rett Syndrome."

96. Anne-Sophie. Lambert et al., "Lower Incidence of Fracture after IV Bisphosphonates in Girls with Rett Syndrome and Severe Bone Fragility," *PLoS ONE* 12, no. 10 (2017): 1–13, https://doi.org/10.1371/journal.pone.0186941.

97. Jenny Downs et al., "Family Satisfaction Following Spinal Fusion in Rett Syndrome," *Developmental Neurorehabilitation* 19, no. 1 (2016): 31–37, https://doi.org/10.3109/17518423.2014.898107; and John T. Killian et al., "Scoliosis in Rett Syndrome: Progression, Comorbidities, and Predictors," *Pediatric Neurology* 70 (2017): 20–25, https://doi.org/10.1016/j.pediatrneurol.2017.01.032.

98. Natalija Krajnc, "Management of Epilepsy in Patients with Rett Syndrome: Perspectives and Considerations," *Therapeutics and Clinical Risk Management* 11 (2015): 925–932, https://doi.org/10.2147/tcrm.s55896.

99. Sharolin Boban et al., "Determinants of Sleep Disturbances in Rett Syndrome: Novel Findings in Relation to Genotype, *American Journal of Medical Genetics Part A* 170, no. 9 (2016): 2,292–2,300, https://doi.org/10.1002/ajmg.a.37784.

100. Anna Urbanowicz et al., "Parental Perspectives on the Communication Abilities of Their Daughters with Rett Syndrome," *Developmental Neurorehabilitation* 19, no. 1 (2016): 17–25, https://doi.org/10.3109/17518423.2013.879940.

101. Urbanowicz et al., "Parental Perspectives on the Communication Abilities of Their Daughters with Rett Syndrome," 19.

102. Urbanowicz et al., "Parental Perspectives on the Communication Abilities of Their Daughters with Rett Syndrome."

103. Vera Munde, Carla Vlaskamp, and A. ter Haar, "Social-Emotional Instability in Individuals with Rett Syndrome: Parents Experiences with Second Stage Behaviour," *Journal of Intellectual Disability Research* 60, no. 1 (2016): 43–53, https://doi.org/10.1111/jir.12233.

104. Susan A. Rose et al., "Sustained Attention in the Face of Distractors: A Study of Children with Rett Syndrome," *Neuropsychology* 31, no. 4 (2017): 403–410, https://doi.org/10.1037/neu0000369.

105. US Department of Health and Human Services, Centers for Disease Control and Prevention, "Sickle Cell Disease (SCD)," August 31, 2016, retrieved December 16, 2017, https://www.cdc.gov/ncbddd/sicklecell/data.html.

106. US Department of Health and Human Services, National Institutes of Health, National Heart, Lung, and Blood Institute, "Sickle Cell Disease: Risk Factors," retrieved December 16, 2017, https://www.nhlbi.nih.gov/health-topics/sickle-cell-disease.

107. David G. Bundy et al., "Urgency of Emergency Department Visits by Children with Sickle Cell Disease: A Comparison of 3 Chronic Conditions," *Academic Pediatrics* 11, no. 4 (2011): 333–341, https://doi.org/10.1016/j.acap.2011.04.006.

108. Mark T. Gladwin, "Cardiovascular Complications and Risk of Death in Sickle-Cell Disease," *The Lancet* 387, no. 10,037 (2016): 2,565–2,574, https://doi.org/10.1016/s0140-6736(16)00647-4.

109. Gladwin, "Cardiovascular Complications and Risk of Death in Sickle-Cell Disease."

110. Steven H. Yale, Nilton Nagib, and Teresa Guthrie, "Approach to the Vaso-Occlusive Crisis in Adults with Sickle Cell Disease," *American Family Physician* 61, no. 5 (2000): 1,349–1,356.

111. Yale, Nagib, and Guthrie, "Approach to the Vaso-Occlusive Crisis in Adults with Sickle Cell Disease."

112. Yale, Nagib, and Guthrie, "Approach to the Vaso-Occlusive Crisis in Adults with Sickle Cell Disease"; Amanda M. Brandow et al., "Patients with Sickle Cell Disease Have Increased Sensitivity to Cold and Heat," *American Journal of Hematology* 88, no. 1 (2012): 37–43, https://doi.org/10.1002/ajh.23341; and Patjanaporn Chalacheva et al., "Biophysical Markers of the Peripheral Vasoconstriction Response to Pain in Sickle Cell Disease," *PLoS ONE* 12, no. 5 (2017): 1–16, https://doi.org/10.1371/journal.pone.0178353.

113. Yale, Nagib, and Guthrie, "Approach to the Vaso-Occlusive Crisis in Adults with Sickle Cell Disease."

114. Susumu Inoue et al., "Pain Management Trend of Vaso-Occlusive Crisis (VOC) at a Community Hospital Emergency Department (ED) for Patients with Sickle Cell Disease," *Annals of Hematology* 95, no. 2 (2016): 221–225, https://doi.org/10.1007/s00277-015-2558-x.

115. Inoue et al., "Pain Management Trend of Vaso-Occlusive Crisis (VOC) at a Community Hospital Emergency Department (ED) for Patients with Sickle Cell Disease."

116. Nadine Matthie and Coretta Jenerette, "Sickle Cell Disease in Adults: Developing an Appropriate Care Plan," *Clinical Journal of Oncology Nursing* 19, no. 5 (2015): 562–567, https://doi.org/10.1188/15.cjon.562-567.

117. Matthie and Jenerette, "Sickle Cell Disease in Adults," 565.

118. Matthie and Jenerette, "Sickle Cell Disease in Adults."

119. J. Levenson, "Psychiatric Issues in Adults with Sickle Cell Disease," *Primary Psychiatry* 15, no. 5 (2008): 45–49; and Yale, Nagib, and Guthrie, "Approach to the Vaso-Occlusive Crisis in Adults with Sickle Cell Disease."

120. Mayo Clinic, "Anemia," August 8, 2017, retrieved July 3, 2018, https://www.mayoclinic.org/diseases-conditions/anemia/symptoms-causes/syc-20351360; and William C. Shiel, "Sickle Cell Disease," September 7, 2016, retrieved July 3, 2018, https://www.medicinenet.com/sickle_cell/article.htm#sickle_cell_anemia_scd_facts.

121. Jo Howard et al., "Guideline on the Management of Acute Chest Syndrome in Sickle Cell Disease," *British Journal of Haematology* 169, no. 4 (2015): 492–505, https://doi.org/10.1111/bjh.13348.

122. Howard et al., "Guideline on the Management of Acute Chest Syndrome in Sickle Cell Disease," 493.

123. Howard et al., "Guideline on the Management of Acute Chest Syndrome in Sickle Cell Disease."

124. Howard et al., "Guideline on the Management of Acute Chest Syndrome in Sickle Cell Disease."

125. Howard et al., "Guideline on the Management of Acute Chest Syndrome in Sickle Cell Disease."

126. Courtney Lawrence and Jennifer Webb, "Sickle Cell Disease and Stroke: Diagnosis and Management," *Current Neurology and Neuroscience Reports* 16, no. 3 (2016): https://doi.org/10.1007/s11910-016-0622-0.

127. Olubusola B. Oluwole et al., "Cognitive Functioning in Children from Nigeria with Sickle Cell Anemia," *Pediatric Blood & Cancer* 63, no. 11 (2016): 1,990–1,997, https://doi.org/10.1002/pbc.26126.

128. Oluwole et al., "Cognitive Functioning in Children from Nigeria with Sickle Cell Anemia," 1,990.

129. M. S. Islam and P. Anoop, "Current Concepts in the Management of Stroke in Children with Sickle Cell Disease," *Child's Nervous System* 27, no. 7 (2011): 1,037–1,043, https://doi.org/10.1007/s00381-011-1394-0.

130. Islam and Anoop, "Current Concepts in the Management of Stroke in Children with Sickle Cell Disease," 1,037.

131. Lawrence and Webb, "Sickle Cell Disease and Stroke: Diagnosis and Management."

132. Lawrence and Webb, "Sickle Cell Disease and Stroke: Diagnosis and Management."

133. Lawrence and Webb, "Sickle Cell Disease and Stroke: Diagnosis and Management."

134. Gladwin, "Cardiovascular Complications and Risk of Death in Sickle-Cell Disease"; Newton Nunes de Lima-Filho et al., "Exercise-Induced Abnormal Increase of Systolic Pulmonary Artery Pressure in Adult Patients with Sickle Cell Anemia: An Exercise Stress Echocardiography Study," *Echocardiography* 33, no. 12 (2014): 1,880–1,890, https://doi.org/10.1111/echo.12853; D. Alem Mehari et al., "Mortality in Adults with Sickle Cell Disease and Pulmonary Hypertension," *Journal of the American Medical Association* 307, no. 12 (2012): 1,254–1,256, https://doi.org/10.1001/jama.2012.358; and Shoaib Alam and Gregory J. Kato, "Sickle Cell Disease-Associated Pulmonary Hypertension: The Effect of Anemia and High Cardiac Output," *Pulmonary Hypertension* 2, no. 2 (2011): 45–59.

135. Mark T. Gladwin and Vadana Sachdev, "Cardiovascular Abnormalities in Sickle Cell Disease," *Journal of the American College of Cardiology* 59, no. 13 (2012): 1,123–1,133, https://doi.org/10.1016/j.jacc.2011.10.900.

136. Gladwin and Sachdev, "Cardiovascular Abnormalities in Sickle Cell Disease."

137. Gladwin and Sachdev, "Cardiovascular Abnormalities in Sickle Cell Disease"; Bharathi Upadhya et al., "Prolongation of QTc Intervals and Risk of Death among Patients with Sickle Cell Disease," *European Journal of Haematology* 91, no. 2 (2013): 170–178, https://doi.org/10.1111/ejh.12127; Julia H. Indik et al., "Associations of Prolonged QTc in Sickle Cell Disease," *PLoS ONE* 11, no. 10 (2016): 1–11, https://doi.org/10.1371/journal.pone.0164526; and Gladwin, "Cardiovascular Complications and Risk of Death in Sickle-Cell Disease."

138. R. L. Woosley et al., *QTdrugs List*, www.CredibleMeds.org (Oro Valley, AZ: AZCERT, Inc., 2017).

139. P. Cannizzo, "Sickle Cell Retinopathy," *Capsula Eburnea* 5, no. 4 (2010): 15–22; and A. O. Fadugbagbe et al., "Ocular Manifestations of Sickle Cell Disease," *Annals of Tropical Paediatrics* 30, no. 1 (2010): 19–26, https://doi.org/10.1179/146532810x12637745451870.

140. F. Traina et al., "Chronic Liver Abnormalities in Sickle Cell Disease: A Clinicopathological Study in 70 Living Patients," *Acta Haematologica* 118, no. 3 (2007): 129–135, https://doi.org/10.1159/000107744.

141. Brandi Dupervil et al., "Emergency Department Visits and Inpatient Admissions Associated with Priapism among Males with Sickle Cell Disease in the United States, 2006–2010," *PLoS ONE* 11, no. 4 (2016), 1–9, https://doi.org/10.1371/journal.pone.0153257.

142. Kizzy-Clara Cita et al., "Men with Sickle Cell Anemia and Priapism Exhibit Increased Hemolytic Rate, Decreased Red Blood Cell Deformability and Increased Red Blood Cell Aggregate Strength," *PLoS ONE* 11, no. 5 (2016): 1–10, https://doi.org/10.1371/journal.pone.0154866.

143. Dupervil et al., "Emergency Department Visits and Inpatient Admissions Associated with Priapism among Males with Sickle Cell Disease in the United States, 2006–2010"; and Howard et al., "Guideline on the Management of Acute Chest Syndrome in Sickle Cell Disease."

144. Raquel Aves Martins et al., "Cholelithiasis and Its Complications in Sickle Cell Disease in a University Hospital," *Revista Brasileira de Hematologia e Hemoterapia* 39, no. 1 (2017): 28–31, https://doi.org/10.1016/j.bjhh.2016.09.009.

145. R. Grant Steen et al., "Cognitive Deficits in Children with Sickle Cell Disease," *Journal of Child Neurology* 20, no. 2 (2005): 102–107, https://doi.org/10.1177/08830738050200020301.

146. Steen et al., "Cognitive Deficits in Children with Sickle Cell Disease," 104.

147. Jeffrey Schatz and Catherine B. McClellan, "Sickle Cell Disease as a Neurodevelopmental Disorder," *Mental Retardation and Developmental Disabilities Research Reviews*, Special Issue: *Developmental Disability in Chronic Disease*, 12, no. 3 (2006): 200–207, https://doi.org/10.1002/mrdd.20115.

148. Oluwole et al., "Cognitive Functioning in Children from Nigeria with Sickle Cell Anemia"; Gauthamen Rajendran et al., "Cognitive Functions and Psychological Problems in Children with Sickle Cell Anemia," *Indian Pediatrics* 53, no. 6 (2016): 485–488, https://doi.org/10.1007/s13312-016-0877-1; Kelsey E. Smith and Jeffrey Schatz, "Working Memory in Children with Neurocognitive Effects from Sickle Cell Disease: Contributions of the Central Executive and Processing Speed," *Developmental Neuropsychology* 41, no. 4 (2016): 231–244, https://doi.org/10.1080/87565641.2016.1238474; and Samantha Nunes et al., "Comprehensive Neuropsychological Evaluation of Children and Adolescents with Sickle Cell Anemia: A Hospital-Based Sample," *Revista Brasileira de Hematologia e Hemoterapia* 39, no. 1 (2017): 32–39, https://doi.org/10.1016/j.bjhh.2016.09.004.

149. Levenson, "Psychiatric Issues in Adults with Sickle Cell Disease."

150. Yale, Nagib, and Guthrie, "Approach to the Vaso-Occlusive Crisis in Adults with Sickle Cell Disease."

151. Howard et al., "Guideline on the Management of Acute Chest Syndrome in Sickle Cell Disease."

152. Yale, Nagib, and Guthrie, "Approach to the Vaso-Occlusive Crisis in Adults with Sickle Cell Disease."

153. Howard et al., "Guideline on the Management of Acute Chest Syndrome in Sickle Cell Disease."

154. Woosley et al., *QTdrugs List.*

155. Joanna L. Marco and Christine L. Chhakchhuak, "Complications of Systemic Lupus Erythematosus in the Emergency Department," *Emergency Medicine* 50, no. 1 (2018): 6–16, https://doi.org/10.12788/emed.2018.0075.

156. US Department of Health and Human Services, Centers for Disease Control and Prevention, "Lupus," January 8, 2018, retrieved March 3, 2018, https://www.cdc.gov/lupus/facts/detailed.html.

157. Angela Nicklin and Roger W. Byard, "Lethal Manifestations of Systemic Lupus Erythematosus in a Forensic Context," *Journal of Forensic Sciences* 56, no. 2 (2011): 423–428, https://doi.org/10.1111/j.1556-4029.2010.01683.x.

158. Robert Ta, Romulo Celli, and A. Brian West, "Diffuse Alveolar Hemorrhage in Systemic Lupus Erythematosus: Histopathologic Features and Clinical Correlations," *Case Reports in Pathology* 2017 (2017): 1–6, https://doi.org/10.1155/2017/1936282; Reshma M. Khan et al., "Embolic Stroke as the Initial Manifestation of Systemic Lupus Erythematosus," *Case Reports in Rheumatology* 2015 (2015): 1–5, https://doi.org/10.1155/2015/373201; and Ping-Yuan Chen et al., "Systemic Lupus Erythematosus Presenting with Cardiac Symptoms," *American Journal of Emergency Medicine* 32, no. 9 (2014): 1,117–1,119, https://doi.org/10.1016/j.ajem.2014.06.036.

159. Jiri Vymetal et al., "Emergency Situations in Rheumatology with a Focus on Systemic Autoimmune Diseases," *Biomedical Papers* 160, no. 1 (2016): 20–29, https://doi.org/10.5507/bp.2016.002.

160. Chen et al., "Systemic Lupus Erythematosus Presenting with Cardiac Symptoms."

161. Masoom Modi et al., "Chest Pain in Lupus Patients: The Emergency Department Experience," *Clinical Rheumatology* 34, no. 11 (2015): 1,969–1,973, https://doi.org/10.1007/s10067-015-2948-4.

162. Chen et al., "Systemic Lupus Erythematosus Presenting with Cardiac Symptoms."

163. Modi et al., "Chest Pain in Lupus Patients: The Emergency Department Experience."

164. Modi et al., "Chest Pain in Lupus Patients: The Emergency Department Experience."

165. Marco and Chhakchhuak, "Complications of Systemic Lupus Erythematosus in the Emergency Department."

166. Vymetal et al., "Emergency Situations in Rheumatology with a Focus on Systemic Autoimmune Diseases"; and Marco and Chhakchhuak, "Complications of Systemic Lupus Erythematosus in the Emergency Department."

167. Vymetal et al., "Emergency Situations in Rheumatology with a Focus on Systemic Autoimmune Diseases"; and Marco and Chhakchhuak, "Complications of Systemic Lupus Erythematosus in the Emergency Department."

168. Vymetal et al., "Emergency Situations in Rheumatology with a Focus on Systemic Autoimmune Diseases"; and Marco and Chhakchhuak, "Complications of Systemic Lupus Erythematosus in the Emergency Department."

169. Suzanne R. Steinbaum, "Pulmonary Arterial Hypertension," WebMD.com, February 20, 2017, retrieved March 3, 2018, https://www.webmd.com/lung/pulmonary-arterial-hypertension#1.

170. Yi Chen et al., "Severe Pulmonary Arterial Hypertension Secondary to Lupus in the Emergency Department: Proactive Intense Care Associated with a Better Short-Term Survival," *International Journal of Rheumatic Diseases* 18, no. 3 (2015): 331–335. https://doi.org/10.1111/1756-185x.12409.

171. Chen et al., "Severe Pulmonary Arterial Hypertension Secondary to Lupus in the Emergency Department."

172. Marco and Chhakchhuak, "Complications of Systemic Lupus Erythematosus in the Emergency Department."

173. Marco and Chhakchhuak, "Complications of Systemic Lupus Erythematosus in the Emergency Department."

174. Marco and Chhakchhuak, "Complications of Systemic Lupus Erythematosus in the Emergency Department."

175. Marco and Chhakchhuak, "Complications of Systemic Lupus Erythematosus in the Emergency Department."

176. Marco and Chhakchhuak, "Complications of Systemic Lupus Erythematosus in the Emergency Department"; and Vymetal et al., "Emergency Situations in Rheumatology with a Focus on Systemic Autoimmune Diseases."

177. Marco and Chhakchhuak, "Complications of Systemic Lupus Erythematosus in the Emergency Department"; and Vymetal et al., "Emergency Situations in Rheumatology with a Focus on Systemic Autoimmune Diseases."

178. Elisheva Pokroy-Shapira, Ilana Gelernter, and Yair Molad, "Evolution of Chronic Kidney Disease in Patients with Systemic Lupus Erythematosus over a Long-Period Follow-up: A Single-Center Inception Cohort Study," *Clinical Rheumatology* 33, no. 5 (2014): 649–657, https://doi.org/10.1007/s10067-014-2527-0; and Marco and Chhakchhuak, "Complications of Systemic Lupus Erythematosus in the Emergency Department."

179. Pokroy-Shapira, Gelernter, and Molad, "Evolution of Chronic Kidney Disease in Patients with Systemic Lupus Erythematosus over a Long-Period Follow-up."

180. Marco and Chhakchhuak, "Complications of Systemic Lupus Erythematosus in the Emergency Department."

181. Pokroy-Shapira, Gelernter, and Molad, "Evolution of Chronic Kidney Disease in Patients with Systemic Lupus Erythematosus over a Long-Period Follow-up."

182. Carolina G. Lins and Mittermayer B. Santiago, "Ultrasound Evaluation of Joints in Systemic Lupus Erythematosus: A Systematic Review," *European Radiology* 25, no. 9 (2015): 2,688–2,692, https://doi.org/10.1007/s00330-015-3670-y.

183. Annamaria Iagnocco et al., "Ultrasound Evaluation of Hand, Wrist, and Foot Joint Synovitis in Systemic Lupus Erythematosus," *Rheumatology* 53, no. 3 (2014): 465–472, https://doi.org/10.1093/rheumatology/ket3761.

184. Sau Mei Tse and Chi Chiu Mok, "Time Trend and Risk Factors of Avascular Bone Necrosis in Patients with Systemic Lupus Erythematosus," *Lupus* 26, no. 7 (2017): 715–722, https://doi.org/10.1177/0961203316676384; and D. D. Gladman et al., "Osteonecrosis in SLE: Prevalence, Patterns, Outcomes and Predictors," Lupus 27, no. 1 (2018): 76–81, https://doi.org/10.1177/0961203317711012.

185. Gladman et al., "Osteonecrosis in SLE: Prevalence, Patterns, Outcomes and Predictors."

186. D. Zelman, "Avascular Necrosis (Osteonecrosis)," WebMD.com, September 1, 2016, retrieved March 10, 2018, https://www.webmd.com/arthritis/avascular-necrosis-osteonecrosis-symptoms-treatments#1.

187. Gladman et al., "Osteonecrosis in SLE: Prevalence, Patterns, Outcomes and Predictors."

188. Gladman et al., "Osteonecrosis in SLE: Prevalence, Patterns, Outcomes and Predictors."

189. Marco and Chhakchhuak, "Complications of Systemic Lupus Erythematosus in the Emergency Department."

190. Marco and Chhakchhuak, "Complications of Systemic Lupus Erythematosus in the Emergency Department."

191. C. Naveau and F. A. Houssiau, "Pneumococcal Sepsis in Patients with Systemic Lupus Erythematosus," *Lupus* 14, no. 11 (2005): 903–906, https://doi.org/10.1191/0961203305lu2242xx.

192. O. Barrett et al., "Mortality Due to Sepsis in Patients with Systemic Lupus Erythematosus and Rheumatoid Arthritis," *Israel Medical Association Journal* 16, no. 10 (2014): 634–635.

193. Nicklin and Byard, "Lethal Manifestations of Systemic Lupus Erythematosus in a Forensic Context."

194. Nicklin and Byard, Lethal Manifestations of Systemic Lupus Erythematosus in a Forensic Context."

195. H. Timlin and M. Petri, "Transient Ischemic Attack and Stroke in Systemic Lupus Erythematosus," *Lupus* 22, no. 12 (2013): 1,251–1,258, https://doi.org/10.1177/0961203313497416; and L. C. D. de Amorim, F. M. Maia, and C. E. M. Rodrigues, "Stroke in Systemic Lupus Erythematosus and Antiphospholipid Syndrome: Risk Factors, Clinical Manifestations, Neuroimaging, and Treatment," *Lupus* 26, no. 5 (2017): 529–536, https://doi.org/10.1177/0961203316688784.

196. Timlin and Petri, "Transient Ischemic Attack and Stroke in Systemic Lupus Erythematosus."

197. Bik Ling Man, Chi Chiu Mok, and Yat Pang Fu, "Neuro-Ophthalmologic Manifestations of Systemic Lupus Erythematosus: A Systematic Review," *International Journal of Rheumatic Diseases* 17, no. 5 (2014): 494–501, https://doi.org/10.1111/1756-185x.12337.

198. Marco and Chhakchhuak, "Complications of Systemic Lupus Erythematosus in the Emergency Department"; Vymetal et al., "Emergency Situations in Rheumatology with a Focus on Systemic Autoimmune Diseases"; and John G. Hanly et al., "Mood Disorders in Systemic Lupus Erythematosus," *Arthritis & Rheumatology* 67 no. 7 (2015): 1,837–1,847, https://doi.org/10.1002/art.39111.

199. Marta Vadacca et al., "Alexithymia, Mood States and Pain Experience in Systemic Lupus Erythematosus and Rheumatoid Arthritis," *Clinical Rheumatology* 33, no. 10 (2014): 1,443–1,450, https://doi.org/10.1007/s10067-014-2593-3.

200. Hanly, "Mood Disorders in Systemic Lupus Erythematosus."

201. E. Waldheim et al., "Health-Related Quality of Life, Fatigue and Mood in Patients with SLE and High Levels of Pain Compared to Controls and Patients with Low Levels of Pain, *Lupus* 22, no. 11 (2013): 1,118–1,127, https://doi.org/10.1177/0961203313502109.

202. Faruk Uguz et al., "Mood, Anxiety and Personality Disorders in Patients with Systemic Lupus Erythematosus," *Comprehensive Psychiatry* 54, no. 4 (2013): 341–345, https://doi.org/10.1016/j.comppsych.2012.10.003.

203. N. Alsowaida et al., "Medication Adherence, Depression and Disease Activity among Patients with Systemic Lupus Erythematosus," *Lupus* 27, no. 2 (2018): 327–332, https://doi.org/10.1177/0961203317725585.

204. Vadacca et al., "Alexithymia, Mood States and Pain Experience in Systemic Lupus Erythematosus and Rheumatoid Arthritis."

205. Vadacca et al., "Alexithymia, Mood States and Pain Experience in Systemic Lupus Erythematosus and Rheumatoid Arthritis."

206. Jill P. Buyon et al., "Predictors of Pregnancy Outcomes in Patients with Lupus: A Cohort Study," *Annals of Internal Medicine* 163, no. 3 (2015): 143–164, https://doi.org/10.7326/M14-2235.

207. Tomasz Hawro et al., "Intractable Headaches, Ischemic Stroke, and Seizures Are Linked to the Presence of Anti-β2GPI Antibodies in Patients with Systemic Lupus Erythematosus," *PLoS ONE* 10, no. 3 (2015): 1–14, https://doi.org/10.1371/journal.pone.0119911; Marco and Chhakchhuak, "Complications of Systemic Lupus Erythematosus in the Emergency Department"; and Vymetal et al., "Emergency Situations in Rheumatology with a Focus on Systemic Autoimmune Diseases."

208. J. L. Huggins, M. J. Holland, and H. I. Brunner, "Organ Involvement Other than Lupus Nephritis in Childhood-Onset Systemic Lupus Erythematosus," *Lupus* 25, no. 8 (2016): 857–863, https://doi.org/10.1177/0961203316644339.

209. Modi et al., "Chest Pain in Lupus Patients: The Emergency Department Experience."

About the Author

Katherine Koch, PhD, is an associate professor of educational studies at St. Mary's College of Maryland. She teaches courses in special education, learning disabilities, behavior disabilities, and research design. Prior to this she was an elementary school special education teacher. Dr. Koch's research focuses on ways to create a more inclusive environment for people with disabilities both in the schools and in the community. As a 911 paramedic, she also writes and speaks on the intersection of disability and prehospital emergency medicine, looking at ways to facilitate the assessment and treatment of people with disabilities in medical and trauma emergencies.

Index